Fatburners

By
George L. Redmon, Ph.D., N.D.

To Lorri
Thanks For
All you Help!"
Dr George

Natural Born Fatburners

George L. Redmon, Ph.D., N.D.

Cover design by Dianne Cooper Bridges

Copyright© 2002 Safe Goods Publishing

ISBN 1-884820-68-9
Library of Congress Catalog Card Number 2002106955

Printed in USA

Natural Born Fatburners is not intended as medical advice. It is written solely for informational and educational purposes. Please consult a health professional should the need for one be indicated. Because there is always some risk involved, the author and publisher are not responsible for any adverse effects or consequences resulting from the use of any of the suggestions, preparations or methods described in this book. The publisher does not advocate the use of any particular diet or health program, but believes the information presented in this book should be available to the public.

All listed addresses, phone numbers and fees have been reviewed and updated during production. However the data is subject to change.

Safe Goods Publishing
561 Shunpike Rd.
Sheffield, MA 01257
413-229-7935

The Author

Dr. Redmon was born in Edenton, North Carolina, and has resided most of his life in Philadelphia, PA. He graduated with honors and earned his Bachelor's Degree in Health in 1974 and was honored as a member of Who's Who Among College Students in America. Dr. Redmond is a graduate, of the Clayton College of Natural Health (ND), the American Holistic College of Nutrition (Ph.D) and received his Ph.D in Administration and Management from Walden University.

Dr. Redmon has developed a 20-year career specializing in vitamins and holistic healthcare within the vitamin and natural health care industry. He has served as a Regional and National Education Director for one of the largest retailers of vitamins in the United States. He is a popular guest on many syndicated radio health programs and his articles have appeared in numerous magazines. Dr. Redmon is also the author of *Managing And Preventing Arthritis: The Natural Alternatives* (Hohm Press), *Minerals: What Your Body Really Needs and Why* (Avery), *Managing And Preventing Prostate Disturbances: The Natural Alternatives,* (Hohm Press), *Energy For Life* (Vital Health Publishing), and *Prime Time Sex For Life: The Natural Alternatives* (Kensington Publishers – Summer 2002).

He is a member of the Herbal Healer Academy, an Adjunct Faculty Member (Adult Health Education) with the Washington Township Public School System in Sewell, NJ, and serves as President of the Board of Directors for the Gallery Market East Mall Merchants Associations in Philadelphia, PA.

Dr. Redmon currently resides in Sicklerville, NJ, with his wife Brenda and their son George Jr.

Acknowledgements

I will be forever indebted to Mr. Eric Dettrey and his secretarial support staff for their fine efforts and dedication towards the completion of this book.

I would like to give a special thanks to Mrs. Lorri Fioravanti for her individual and exceptional editorial and copy work, without which this project would have been severely compromised. Thank you Lorri.

As a researcher, I would like to give thanks to the past and present investigators, scientists and healthcare professionals whose diligence and devotion to the preservation of human life, motivates me toward that same cause. I am also sincerely grateful to my editor Ms. Nina Anderson, of Safe Goods Publishing and her colleagues for providing the platform for this topic's review and study.

This author owes a sincere debt of gratitude to my wife Brenda and my son George Jr. for their undying support. Lastly, I would like to acknowledge the following individuals who gave their emotional and intellectual support, which contributed greatly to the completion of this project.

- Ms. Andrea Foster, Director
  The Holistic Resource and
  Referral Network of Houston, TX

- Dr. Barry Persky, Ph.D.
  New York City University
  Department of Education
  New York, NY

- Dr. Pamela Peters, Ph.D.
  Director and Founder
  The Center for Stress Pain and Wellness Management
  Wilmington, DE

- Dr. Marcia B. Steinhauer, Ph.D.
  Department of Health and Human Services
  Walden University
  Minneapolis, MN

Dedication

This book is dedicated to my father, George Redmon Jr., for his devotion, love and guidance. I will be forever grateful.

Table of Contents

Prologue

After years of fading into the background, diet pills are once again exploding with popularity. This trend has caused great reason for concern. Recent studies published in the New England Journal of Medicine have revealed that the use of drugs to reduce appetite (mainly derivatives of fenfluramine) are associated with a profound increase of an often fatal lung disorder called pulmonary hypertension.
-Dr. David Perlmutter, M.D.
The Commons Medical and Surgical Center, Naples, Florida

In February 1996, Josie developed a nagging cough that our family doctor said was bronchitis. It persisted through the summer, and by late August, she was having trouble breathing. Around 12:30 a.m. on November 20th, I got a call from Josie's mother at the intensive care unit. When I arrived, the cardiologist on duty walked up and said, 'I'm sorry, her lungs just gave out on her. She's dead.

-Hallie Levine, "Fen-phen killed my wife," Cosmopolitan, December, 1997

I took care of those people. It was difficult telling them that a transplant may be in their future, and pregnancy may be out of the question, and it is even sadder that this is the result of something that was avoidable.
-Dr. Lewis Ruben, M.D., Top U.S. Expert on Primary Pulmonary Hypertension

We had physicians treating millions of people, [prescribing for them] based on a study with only a [mere] dozen people.
-Dr. Leolutwak, M.D., Endocrinologist and Medical Officer, FDA

Neither the drugs on the market now, nor any that might be available in the future are going to solve the problem of obesity. There are drugs that are helpful, but all of them only produce modest weight loss. All of them have side effects.
-David Allison, Assistant Research Scientist, St. Luke's Roosevelt Hospital Center, NY

While weight loss is the gold standard of success for most people who diet, it is only one of the benefits of a diet and fitness program. Along with weight loss, a reduction in blood pressure, blood glucose levels and blood cholesterol also should be deemed as desirable goals. Additionally, feeling better physically, a sense of increased awareness and responsibility for personal health and increased optimism about life are also important considerations in a weight loss and fat reduction program.
-Mike Hamilton, et al., *Book of Diet and Fitness,* The Duke University Medical Center

Preface

The hype started a little over six years ago, when the FDA approved a new diet pill — the first of its kind in over twenty-three years. The drug was Redux, also known as Dexfenfluramine, or "Fen-Phen." The drug helped maintain higher levels of the brain chemical serotonin, the serenity and pleasure neurotransmitter, also a known appetite suppressant. Launched in June of 1996, the new drug was being prescribed at a rate of about 65,000 new prescriptions per week.

It has taken us a number of decades to realize that there is a connection, interrelationship and correlation of variables that link one's diet to the onset of disease. The host of variables includes, but is not limited to, genetic disposition, mindset and lifestyle. The attitudes and roles of our physicians also play a part in how we think about health issues, since we look to them for answers. Indeed, there are many caring and educated health professionals out there, teaching their patients to eat right and live a healthy lifestyle. Unfortunately, there are also others who simply rely on medication as the answer to the problem. And even though there is a wealth of information regarding the dangers of dieting drugs and wrongful dieting in general, there appears to be a general resurgence of thinking that touts dieting drugs as an answer to America's obesity problem. One of the most insidious paradoxes in all the hoopla surrounding the new diet drugs is that studies show that in many cases:

- the drugs clearly are less effective when tolerance levels are reached;
- many individuals regain all the weight that was lost within months after stopping the drug;
- weight loss with drugs averaged less than 20 pounds in a year as compared to 14 pounds of weight loss for those individuals who took placebos: and
- individuals actually gained weight while on the drugs.

Although the drug "Fen-Phen" is now banned from use, the battle is not over. The financial rewards of this new era of diet drugs seem to outweigh the risks associated with long-term health. Newly refined versions, black market sales and other diet drugs are poised to flood the market place in this new century.

As health care professionals, as well as the general public, we simply cannot ignore the facts that have emerged in reference to the recent deaths or possible long-term residual effects associated with the use of the new breed of diet drugs. As health professionals, as well as you the individual, we must question this new era of "diet drugs" that exhibit lethal ramifications with use. More importantly, however, we should challenge their threat to the current movement of social empowerment, awareness and reliance on participative preventive measures, versus indulgence and dependence on consequent treatment.

In September 1997, the FDA issued a recall of the popular diet drugs, Pondimin (Fenfluramine), and Redux (Dexfenfluramine or "Fen-Phen.") Continued reported cases of possible brain damage and heart-valve abnormalities prompted this action by the Food and Drug Administration. However, this has not prevented the development of new drugs.

Consider the year 2000 introduction of the diet drug Meridia, approved by the Food and Drug Administration (FDA) to be used for the medical management of obesity. This drug carries stiff warnings. As cited in the information bulletin by Knoll Pharmaceutical on Meridia: "Meridia should not be taken by people who have uncontrolled or poorly controlled high blood pressure, due to the possible side effect of substantially increased blood pressure in some patients."

Or take for example, a warning recently issued concerning the practice of combining the diet drug "Phendimetrazine" with Phentermine. Medical professionals are warning physicians that this drug's application is not warranted for use with any other anorexigenic (diet) drugs. (*Please see Appendix A*).

As health care professionals, we must continually ask ourselves, are we becoming mirrored images of the technology that surrounds us? Are we looking for quick fixes and immediate results, without considering the long-term health of those we seek to help?

With all the viable natural supplements and programs that are gaining acceptance, there are ways to address the issues of obesity without drugs. If you are contemplating the use of dieting drugs, please think twice about your decision. Read this book and find out how you can train your body to optimize its metabolism of calories. If you have already been diagnosed as clinically obese or if you suspect that you might be, or if you have other health issues in addition to being overweight, please first consult your physician. And always remember — **You do not have to die to be thin!**
-Dr. George L. Redmon, Ph.D., N.D.

Introduction

Based on current data, Americans are continuously dieting, yet they are getting fatter. As the number of Americans who are considered to be overweight escalates, current medical reasoning seeks to substantiate the need for diet drugs. Dr. David Levitsky, a professor of Nutrition and Psychology at Cornell University, maintains that this new era of diet drugs obscures the true underlying issues. The real issue, he reminds us, is lifestyle. Levitsky argues that the new drugs give people a false sense of security, and a quick fix. He notes, "The new diet drugs undermine the advice we have given for years, such as reducing fat intake, lowering total calorie load, eating more fruits and fiber and exercising."

The federal government plans to change its definition of obesity, skewing the weight requirements lower. It has been estimated that under the new guidelines, based on the Body Mass Index, roughly half of American adults will be considered to be overweight. These new guidelines will make it easier for many Americans to be classified as clinically obese and as such meet certain criteria for use of new diet drugs that are poised to hit the market.

The Purpose of This Book

The goal of *Natural Born Fat Burners* is to introduce you to a new and exciting way to lose weight and to reduce body fat, safely and effectively, without the aid of dangerous diet drugs. *Natural Born Fat Burners* is designed to show you how to develop short-term interchangeable goals that have life-saving implications in your quest to shed unwanted pounds and maintain desired weight levels. After reviewing and putting into practice the programs as outlined here, you will be able to:

- calculate your daily caloric needs;
- "train" your natural fatburning cycles;
- choose and establish a natural fatburning supplement program that suits your individual biochemical profile;
- set up your very own individualized exercise program that is safe and effective;
- understand once and for all the negative consequences of off-and-on dieting;
- determine your individual metabolic capacity;

- set up and self-administer safe and effective internal detox-ification regimens to induce and/or enhance natural fatburning cycles;
- establish contact with various organizations and associations that deal with issues related to weight control and its management;
- double your current energy levels.

The overall goal of *Natural Born Fat Burners* is to show you how to naturally augment normal metabolic cycles without the use of dangerous diet drugs. To give you an overall picture of how you can set up, re-establish or fine-tune your natural fatburning ability for life, this book has been divided into eleven chapters, each one designed to guide you through the learning process in as clear and straightforward a way as possible. Enjoy, be well and keep in touch.

Chapter One

Food: Your Most Prolific Fatburner

The real problem in most cases of obesity begins with how many calories you use while you are not doing anything, not while you are exercising. Basal metabolism (the calories you use at rest under standard conditions) decreases as you get older.

Dr. Lawrence E. Lamb M.D.,
Metabolics: Putting Your Food Energy to Work[1]

By Nature, You're a Fatburning Machine

For all intents and purposes, nature has programmed you to co-exist as one of its major sources of energy. You are an interminable energy factor capable of converting, storing and using energy to carry out life's processes. You are energy personified, capable of great feats. You can convert energy from the food you consume that fuels you and allows you to do muscular work. This process of energy conversion is a reciprocal process between you and nature. Through this dynamic energy flow, not only do obesity researchers know that you can control weight with food by manipulating brain neurotransmitter activity, they also know that by utilizing certain natural foods in various combinations you can recalibrate your body's metabolic rate and become an interminable, never-ending fatburning machine.

According to Dr. Marc Rogers, author of *Stuff Yourself Slim*, scientist now know how to combine nutrients to burn off fat. Certain foods tagged as negative calorie foods, metabolic or catabolic foods, have the capacity to actually increase your basal metabolic rate (BRM), thereby burning more fat while your body is at rest. As cited by Dr. Rogers, these natural fatburning foods stimulate basal metabolism, accounting for nearly 70 percent of the calories your body burns up and utilizes for energy.[2] It is interesting to note that studies have also shown that reducing normal established food intake actually depresses or slows down resting metabolic rates by as much as 45 percent and continues to decline even more with each and every attempt at dieting.[3] Therefore, it is important to eat, to eat plenty and to eat the correct foods for your metabolic type.

13

Metabolism is defined as the chemical processes continuously going on in living organisms. Basal metabolism is the term used to describe the energy the body expends when it is at rest but awake. This is one of the most overlooked aspects of weight control, according to Dr. Lawrence E. Lamb M.D., author of *Metabolics: Putting Your Food Energy To Work*. He suggests that the secret and scientific facts about controlling weight have been around for a long time. Dr. Lamb is a former Professor of Medicine at Baylor University and Chief of Medical Sciences at the School of Aerospace Medicine.

The scientific fact whereby the body uses its own heat to burn up excess calories is known as thermogenesis. This process, first theorized by a researcher from Harvard University in 1967, has been confirmed and re-confirmed by modern day researchers like Dr. Daniel B. Mowrey, Director of Scientific Affairs of Klein-Becker. Dr. Robert E. Kowalski the nationally known author of *The 8-Week Cholesterol Cure,* also reminds us that scientists call this inborn fatburning ability the law of the thermodynamics. Dr. Kowalski says when you take in calories from foods (calories being a measure of energy), your body has the choice of expending calories as energy or storing them as fat. "In the long run," he says, "diets simply don't work. Going on a diet normally implies eventually going off the diet. In the meantime, nothing has happened to change the poor eating habits that led to obesity in the first place." Kowalski continues: "The only way to lose weight permanently is to completely change one's attitude and approaches toward food."[4]

Our approach to maintaining healthy weight levels here in America has been largely misdirected. Dr. Neal Barnard, M.D., a well-known medical professional and author of *Foods That Cause You to Lose Weight: The Negative Calorie Effect,* reminds us that the human body took shape millions of years ago and when we diet or starve ourselves we slow down the rate at which we burn up calories. Dr. Barnard insists that we need to move beyond the out-dated mode of counting calories and limiting portion size. New research has confirmed that the key to weight control is not how much you eat but the kind of foods you consume. This is the basis of the negative calorie or metabolic capacity of foods. Some foods actually *enhance* your metabolism. New research shows that you can actually eat more of these foods and lose weight, maintain healthier cholesterol levels, feel full and retain your energy levels. Consider the following:

• Researchers in Canada at the University of Calgary found that MCT (medium chain triglyceride) oil administered to individuals on a low carbohydrate diet increased the body's ability to burn up body fat while decreasing loss of lean muscle, the body's most prolific fatburning agent. MCT are fats that are not easily stored by the body because of their molecular structure. They are burned up rapidly in the liver as a fuel and stimulate heat production better known as theromogensis, which increases the body's ability to burn up excess fat. MCT oil can be purchased at your local health food store.[5]

• Clinical studies of the effects of soy products over the past several decades show a cause-and-effect relationship to reduced cholesterol levels as well as an increase in HDL (good) ratio to LDL (bad) cholesterol levels.[6]

• Research conducted at the Department of Medicine at the University of Kentucky proved that oat bran significantly lowered LDL cholesterol by 36 percent while increasing HDL levels by 82 percent. As a soluble fiber, it attaches to fat particles and fastens there passing through the digestive tract unabsorbed.[7]

• Researchers from the Diet, Safety and Health Economics Branch of the U.S. Department of Agriculture in Washington, D.C. recently established new guidelines specifically targeting an increase in whole-grain intake. Recommendations include increasing the proportion of persons aged two years and older who consume at least six daily servings of grain products with at least three servings including whole grains.[8]

Unrefined whole grains supply the body with complex carbohydrates that contain fiber. These grains curb appetite, help stabilize blood sugar (discouraging fat storage) and are rich in vitamins, minerals, protein and other protective substances. Examples of whole grains are oats, brown rice, barley, wheat germ, whole wheat, rice bran, oatmeal and unprocessed bran.

Managing Your Life-Long Fatburning Potential

Researchers from the Centers for Disease Control studying the rising trend of obesity in America from 1991 to 1998 concluded that obesity continues to rise at an alarming rate. They found that between the years 1991 and 1998, obesity as defined by a body mass index of over 30kg/m increased from 12.0 to 17.9 percent. This steady increase was found in both males and females in all age groups, races as well as educational and socio-economic status. This study[9] revealed that the largest increases of weight occurred in the following groups of people:

- 18 to 29 years old (7.1% to 12.1%);
- those with some college education (10.6% to 17.8%); and
- individuals of Hispanic ethnicity (11.6% to 20.8%).

To counter this trend, the authors concluded that strategies and programs to control weight must become a much higher public priority. A recent follow-up study found the percentage of increase of obesity is now at 19.8 percent.[10] This study also concluded that:

- 27 percent of U.S. adults do not engage in any physical activity and another 28 percent were sedentary;
- only 24 percent of the adult population consume fruits or vegetables five or more times a week;
- of the patients who were already overweight during regular routine exams, 42.8 percent were further advised to lose weight;
- among individuals engaged in some kind of diet reduction program and exercising at least 150 minutes per week, 17.5% of them were having problems losing and/or maintaining normal weight levels.

Based on current data, America is in a silent but severe epidemic that is spiraling out of control. Additionally, while most of the individuals in America are on some type of diet and exercise program, we as a nation continue to get fatter.

In his book, *Naturally Slim and Powerful,* Dr. Philip Lipetz writes, "Serotonin-enhancing drugs are powerless with a diet that lowers serotonin. The drugs work by making serotonin work more effectively. If there is no serotonin, there is nothing for these drugs to work on. This means that people must eat the proper foods in order for these drugs to work."[11]

According to Dr. Lipetz, many current diet drugs work by altering serotonin. Serotonin is a brain neurotransmitter that helps modulate many functions in the body such as, sleep, mood, food intake, pain tolerance, depression, and food cravings. Serotonin production is directly related to diet with some foods being better than others for producing serotonin. Dieting drugs enhance the effects of serotonin already present but do not actually supply serotonin. Food supplies the ingredients for serotonin production. Serotonin is manufactured in the brain from the amino acid tryptophan, which is produced by protein-rich foods aided by vitamin B_6, B_{12}, folic acid and other nutrients. As quoted by Elizabeth Somer, M.A., R.D., author of *Food and Mood* and a nationally known registered dietician, "Serotonin levels are directly related to the amount of tryptophan in the blood and the availability of these vitamins. That is, as blood and brain levels of tryptophan rise and fall, and as vitamin intake fluctuates between optimal and deficient, so does the level of serotonin."[12]

The above findings were also confirmed by research at the Massachusetts Institute of Technology (MIT) Clinical Research Center, headed by Dr. Judith J. Wurtman, Ph.D. Dr. Wurtman, one of the country's most eminent bio-nutritional researchers, found that eating certain foods at specific times could elevate serotonin levels naturally thus controlling appetite, mood, depression, food cravings and weight. Anti-obesity researchers already know that many of the body's natural mood-elevating appetite suppressants and weight control agents are produced and controlled by the food we eat. In retrospect, contrary to proper belief Xenical, Orilistat, Prozac, Pondimin (Fenfluramine) and other anti-obesity drugs are not "nature's" prescribed weight-loss aids.

Louise Gittleman, M.S., one of the country's most noted nutritionists and author of *Your Body Knows Best*, insists that complex carbohydrates eaten with lean proteins will speed up the metabolic rate and should be an integral part of the slow burners diet. She also cites another reason to make sure there is adequate protein in your diet: protein stimulates the production of glucagons, a hormone that inhibits the fat-storage activity of insulin, which is released by the body when carbohydrates are eaten.[13]

Note: *It is simple carbohydrates like sugar, candy, cakes, pies, cookies, that promote the over-secretion of insulin to offset the rising blood sugar levels.*

According to Ms. Gittleman, lean meats such as chicken, turkey and white fish are also vital to speeding up metabolism. She reasons that this is why (using lean protein and complex carbohydrates) individuals whose metabolic rate is slow have great success on diet programs like Weight Watchers, Lean Bodies and Overeaters Anonymous. Additionally supplying the body with a variety of nutrients is essential to helping the body break down fat. In fact, Udo Erasmus, author of the highly acclaimed *Fats That Heal, Fats That Kill*, states that, "out of the 45 known essential nutrients, at least 29 are involved in fat metabolism."[14]

Dr. Barbara Edelstein, M.D., author of *The Underburner's Diet: How to Rid Your Body of Excess Fat Forever*, says that you can use certain foods to stoke the metabolic furnace. According to

Dr. Edelstein, every food has a specific dynamic action (SDA), which is the amount of energy the body uses to break it down. From her research on obesity, Dr. Edelstein has also found protein to have a most profound capacity to keep the BMR (Basal Metabolic Rate) on high.

Even the famed diet guru Dr. Robert Atkins, M.D., suggests we keep a watchful eye on our metabolism. Dr. Atkins says that not everyone loses weight with the same ease, even on a low carbohydrate diet. He argues that the person who is truly metabolically resistant won't lose much at all without getting more exercise or taking nutritional supplements that help weight loss, or restricting the quantity of food eaten.[15] For those of you who need a little extra help, in Chapter Six, *Natural Born Fatburners,* you will find an array of nutritional supplements that can be utilized safely and effectively to assist you in your fatburning efforts.

The following chapters reveal how to:
1. keep your metabolic rate in overdrive and burn up your calories at a faster rate while enjoying wholesome, fulfilling food;
2. assist your body in maintaining healthy cholesterol levels, losing unwanted pounds and inches, while maintaining fantastic levels of energy; and
3. eat more often, stabilize your blood sugar levels, reduce body fat and control your appetite, while protecting your heart and improving your overall well-being!

---

[1] Lamb, L.E., *Metobolics: Putting Your Food Energy To Work,* New York: Harper and Row, 1974.

[2] Rogers, S., "How the Sick Get Sicker Quicker Without Nutritional Supplements," *Let's Live* 62, No. 1 (Jan, 1994): 44-47.

[3] *Miller, D.S., Parsonage, S., "Resistance to slimming: Adaptation or illusion",* Lancet, 1975: 1: 733.

[4] Kowalski,R.E. The Eight-Week Cholesterol Cure, Harper and Rowe, NY, 1989, p.140.

[5] Dias, V. "Effects of Feeding and Energy Balance in Adult Humans," Metabolism, 1990 (39): 887: 891.

[6] Anderson, J.W., Johnstone, B.M., Cook – Newell, M.E., "Meta-analysis of the effects of soy protein intake on serum lipids", New England Journal of Medicine, 1995 (333): 276-282.

[7] Anderson, J.W., Chen, W.L., "Plant fiber, carbohydrate and lipid (fat) metabolism" American Journal of Clinical Nutrition, 1979 (32): 346-363.

[8] Kantor, L.S., Jayachandran V.,N., Allshouse, J.E., et.al., "Choose a variety of grains daily, especially whole grains: A challenge for consumers," Journal of Nutrition, 2001: 131: 473S-486S.

[9] Mokdad, A. H., Serdula, M.K., Dietz, W.H., et. al., "The Spread of the Obesity Epidemic in the United States, 1991-1998," JAMA 1999 282 (16): 1519-1522.

[10] Mokdad, A.H., Bowman, B.A., Ford, E.S., et. Al., "The continuing Epidemics of Obesity and Diabetes in the United States," JAMA, 2001, 286 (10): 1195-2000.

[11] Lipetz., P. *Naturally Slim and Powerful*, Andrews & McMeel, Kansas City, MO, 1997.

[12] Somer, E., *Food and Mood*, Henry Holt & Co., NY, 1995.

[13] Gittleman, L., *Your Body Knows Best*, Pocket Books, NY, 1996.

[14] Erasmus, U., *Fats That Heal, Fats That Kill*, Designing Health, Menlo Park, CA, 1988, p.10.

[15] Atkins, R.C., *Dr. Atkins New Diet Revolution*, p. 23, New York, NY: Avon Books, 1999.

Chapter Two

Eating To Induce Fatburning

Calories do count. However, if the diet is nutritionally sound, what one eats is not as important as how much is eaten (that is, how many calories are consumed). If a true calorie deficit exists, then weight loss will occur quite independent of the diet's composition.

**Dr. William D. McArdle, Ph.D. and
Dr. John R. Magel, Ph.D.**
Weight Management: Diet And Exercise[1]

As mentioned earlier, the real key to weight loss is the body's ability to burn up calories when it is at rest. The word *thermogensis* literally refers to the body's ability to create heat. It is this natural process, much like turning on your stove or oven, that assists the body in burning off excess calories and is vital to maintaining and or decreasing weight to normal healthy levels. Obesity researchers call substances that stimulate or turn on this process, thermogenic agents. Jump-starting this process can increase your basal or resting metabolic rate, which causes the body's production of noradrenalin to increase. Noradrenalin is a hormone produced by the adrenal glands that among, other things, stimulates the process of lipolysis, a biochemical process of breaking down or dissolving fats.

Scientists have identified foods that actually stimulate metabolism, and, by consuming them, you have what is known as a negative calorie effect. In essence, these foods actually burn up more calories than they add to the body. For example, a piece of pie consisting of 350 calories may need about 100 calories of energy to be digested and broken down by the body. In this case, there will be 250 additional calories that will eventually be stored as body fat. On the other hand, a stalk of celery may need the same number (100 energy calories) to be broken down and digested, resulting in a net loss of 95 energy calories that the body can use to get rid of excess body fat. Ron J. Clark,[2] President of The National Federation of Personal Fitness Trainers, Judy Jameson, author of *Fat Burning Foods and Other Weight Loss Secrets,*[3] along with Porter Shimer and Betty Bianconi, authors of *More Fat Burning Foods,*[4] present us with new evidence on how the body can actually use calories from certain foods to rid the body of excess fat. This plan reduces weight, safely and effectively. Ron J. Clark reminds us that as negative calorie foods are consumed, they not only encourage enzyme production in quantities sufficient enough to not only metabolize (break down) their own calories, but help to breakdown calories from other foods as well. Adding enzyme supplements to your diet takes a tremendous burden off the pancreas, which, if overworked, could become depleted of its ability to produce adequate levels of digestive enzymes. In essence, by consuming more of these negative calorie foods, you can increase your body's metabolic rate, thus burning up calories more efficiently, reduce cholesterol levels and reduce weight slowly and gradually.[5]

This is exactly the affirmation proclaimed by Dr. Ardle and Dr. Magel, both professors in physiology at Queens College of City University of New York. Both healthcare professionals who specialize in the field of fitness, weight management and metabolic control, describe the attributes of a true calorie deficit and its effect on weight loss. It is this aspect that researchers make claims regarding fatburning foods, that result in weight loss, better stabilization of blood sugar, decrease in blood pressure and a host of other positive health benefits. In fact, nutritionist Maureen Keane, a former student and instructor at Bastyr University and author of *The Red Yeast Rice Cholesterol Solution,* advises us to:

- eat more fruits and vegetables;
- have at least one serving of soy foods a day;
- take a balanced vitamin, mineral and antioxidant supplement;
- decrease the amount of junk food you consume; and
- stop eating at fast food restaurants and find a eatery that serves healthier foods.

She claims you would see dramatic changes in your health alone by following this regime[6].

Stephen Twigg, author of *Love Food. . .Lose Weight,* and one of Great Britain's most well-known holistic health practitioners, has served as an advisor and consultant to many prominent British royalty figures, including the late Princess Diana. He suggests that of all the methods of dieting you could choose, combining and rotating the right foods fulfills virtually all the essentials of the perfect diet.[7] Dr. Martin Katahn, Ph.D., well-known author and obesity researcher, says that the rotation form of dieting can in many cases, result in up to one pound per day in lost weight. According to

Dr. Katahn, fresh vegetables can be consumed in unlimited quantities ensuring that you never leave the table hungry. He also asks you to remember: "If you will just continue to substitute fresh fruit (any fruit) about 60 or 70 percent of the time, when you might ordinarily eat high-calorie snacks or desserts after you reach your desirable weight, you will be taking a giant step toward permanent weight management."[8]

Rotating Foods To Stimulate Fatburning

Dr. Barbara F. Edelstein, M.D., author of *The Underburners Diet: How to Rid Your Body of Excess Fat Forever,* in her early research on weight disorders, formulated a simple eating program for individuals cited as <u>underburners</u>. The formula consisted of consuming daily.[9]

• two proteins
• one-and-a-half servings of grains or starches
• three fruit servings
• six vegetables
• one dairy product
• vitamin and mineral formula
• one tablespoon of unprocessed bran
• six eight-ounce glasses of water

She also identified what she called "fifty of the best diet foods." According to Dr. Edelstein, specific diets come and go, while it is the foods themselves that create a successful weight-loss program. She found that the best way to control weight permanently is to eat more fatburning foods while rotating them with other specific food categories. This point is very important! Her program ensures that you receive some nutrients from all of the food groups, but a majority from those foods that contain fiber, protein, and come from whole unprocessed food sources.[10]

Your Fatburning Food Plan

While there are many different foods and variations that can help you maintain normal weight levels, it is important to have some idea of the categories and the types of food which support the metabolic processes. We will begin by listing some of the fatburning foods. According to Dr. Neal Barnard, author of *Foods That Cause You To Lose Weight*, many of these foods can be eaten in generous portions without excessive weight gain.[11]

Generally fat-burning foods:

- corn
- rice
- potatoes
- lettuce
- broccoli
- carrots
- black beans
- lentils
- spinach
- pineapple
- celery
- peas
- cauliflower
- cabbage
- oatmeal
- oranges
- apples
- grapefruit
- kidney beans

My top 15 favorites are:

- raw nuts & seeds
- brown rice
- apple cider vinegar
- green leafy vegetables
- whole unprocessed grains
- melons (all)
- olive oil
- navy beans
- cucumbers
- tomatoes
- water
- oatmeal
- tuna
- pink salmon
- yams

Categorizing Your Fatburning Foods

While the list above represents only a small portion of possible fatburning foods, you may want to start with ten to fifteen different types of foods. Slowly replace your current food combinations with these fatburners. Additionally, by rotating the food combinations you can slowly shift your metabolic rate from park to overdrive. A similar method is proposed by Stephen Twigg, who asks his clients to develop a master plan for a daily menu. The idea is to build confidence and have some sort of roadmap. This is not a diet; it is a way to get you to eat those fatburning foods you love. This way you are in control. Use the proposed guidelines as expressed by Dr. Edelstein on the previous page. Do not be concerned about the portion size. Just consume many of your higher calorie foods, such as milk, dairy and meat during mid-day, and not your evening meal.

Make yourself a chart similar to the example below:

Feed Your Machine	First Choice	Second Choice
Breakfast		
Morning Snack		
Lunch		
Dinner		

Which foods do you start out with? In Chapter Five, *Winning Without Diet Drugs* you will find listed 100 of the top foods that can help you keep your metabolic fires burning, even when at rest.

In 1976, research from the Institute for Behavioral Education in King of Prussia Pennsylvania, confirmed that individuals could lose weight safely and effectively by eating. Drs Henry A. Jordan, M.D., professor of Clinical Psychology at the University of Pennsylvania School of Medicine and Leonard S. Levitz, Ph.D., co-director of the Institute, formulated what was known as *The Behavioral Control Diet*. This program, which had been in existence for five years, was considered one of the most successful programs in the field of obesity research. Its key lay in balancing the amount of calories vs. activity to maintain weight or lose weight, focusing on behavior modifications and eating patterns versus pure calorie control. For example, these researchers found that many people tend to eat for the following reasons:[12]

- food is simply available
- out of frustration
- to be sociable
- to relieve tension
- out of boredom
- out of tradition

These researchers insisted that changes in lifestyle and inappropriate eating patterns were the real key to weight management and loss. A similar notion has re-emerged as Linda Omichinski, R.D. and Heather W. Hildebrand, R.N., authors of *Tailoring Your Taste*, suggest that for long-term weight management it is best to throw away your calculator. Their program centers on having the individual slowly adjust their eating habits and food preferences, thereby gradually reducing fat, sugar and excessive salt from their diet. They stress the importance of feeling that any change toward more healthful eating is progress. Research by Dr. Pamela Peeke, M.D., M.P.H., an assistant professor of medicine at the University of Maryland School of Medicine in Baltimore suggests/confirms that cravings for fatty foods during stressful episodes may be a biological impulse. They suggest that, while you focus on foods that you like with the following rules:

- 2/3 to 3/4 of the food on your plate consists of complex carbohydrates and fiber (bread, rice, pasta, fruits and vegetables);
- 1/3 to 1/4 of the meal contains protein (meat, seafood, poultry eggs, cheese, peanut butter, legumes, etc.);
- Eat regularly, every three to six hours;
- Develop a plan of healthful foods you're willing to try purely for health, gradually exchanging them for less desirable unhealthy fatty foods.

Note: *In this book, we have recommended 101 of the top fatburning foods to select from. This change should be done progressively, moving toward long-term weight control and management, versus radical short-term changes and repeated cycles of yo-yo dieting.*

The Columbia University Eating Plan

So far we have focused on eating and not dieting to keep our metabolic rate on high. Jane Brody, the nationally known personal health columnist for the *New York Times*, also suggest eating as a means to long- term weight control. According to Ms. Brody,[13] you can construct a weight-loss menu plan that does not lock you into a limited number of foods or restrict you to foods you don't especially like. She cites several of the 100 fatburning foods we list later, as identified by the Institute of Human Nutrition at Columbia University. Ms. Brody advises that the portion sizes for many of these foods should be kept to ½ cup cooked or one cup in their raw state.

Researchers devised portion amounts of various foods and their ability to assist in weight maintenance or weight loss. By using their guidelines you need not worry about counting calories. The type of food, balance of calories and correct portions that will gently stroke your metabolic fires, have been established for you. The idea is to eat generous portions of these fatburning foods. The daily portion guide listed below will yield the approximate calorie levels indicated.[14] Free foods that can be eaten in unlimited quantities are the foods as described earlier by Dr. Neal Barnard, author of *Foods That Cause you to Lose Weight.*

Calories	1,000	1,200	1,500	1,800
Free foods	Unlimited	Unlimited	Unlimited	Unlimited
Vegetables	2	2	2	2
Fruits	3	3	3	3
Starches	3	5	7	9
Proteins	6	6	7	7
Milk	2	2	2	3
Fats	2	2	6	7

Switching Your Metabolic Rate to Fast Forward

As you begin rotating many of the fatburning foods into your master meal plan, you will be well on your way to eventually completing the most important part of your overall weight-management and fat-loss plan. Your natural fatburning mechanisms that have been dormant will in all intents and purposes be fired up. Give yourself time and enjoy your new food choices, as you begin to discover the real joy of eating and why obesity researchers contend that you actually control and can manipulate your life-long fatburning potential.

Before you can move forward and have any long-term success at controlling your weight, it is imperative that you understand that food is actually your most prolific fatburner. Learning how to use it properly is the most important part of any weight-management program. Your natural fatburning furnaces are run by and maintained by the foods you consume. You can, for all intents and purposes, literally turn off and/or depress your metabolic or natural fatburning capabilities by going on restrictive diets. We will, in the chapters that follow, explore dieting and its negative effects on your metabolic capabilities. Additionally, we will take a look at the importance of exercise, as well as the dangers of diet drugs and natural supplements that are gaining worldwide acceptance as viable alternatives. Finally, we also shall review the concept of toxemia, weight gain and other fatburning food choices, as well as organizations and other health-related institutions that can help you reach your weight and fat loss goals safely, naturally and effectively.

[1] Bland Jeffrey, editor, *Medical Applications of Clinical Nutrition*, Keats Publishing, New Canaan, CT, 1983, p.99-132.

[2] President of The National Federation of Personal Fitness Trainers, Lafayette Indiana.

[3] Jameson, Judy, *Fat Burning Foods and Other Weight Loss Secrets* McGraw Hill, 1996.

[4] Shimer, Porter, Bianconi. Betty, *More Fat Burning Foods,* NTC /Contemporary Publishing, 1998.

[5] Clark R.J., "Negative Calorie Foods," Personal Trainer Magazine, Lafeyette IN, 1999. (Article can be found at www.nfpt.com/library/articles/pstwkt.html).

[6] Keane, M., *The Red Yeast Rice Cholesterol Solution*, Adams Media Corporation, Holbrook, MA, 1999.

[7] Twigg, S., *Love Food. . .Lose Weight,* Penguin Publishing, New York, NY, 1997.

[8] Katahn, M., *The Rotation Diet*, Bantam Books, NY, 1986.

[9] Edelstein, B., The Underburner's Diet: How To Rid Your Body of Excess -Fat Forever, New York: MacMillan Publishing, 1987.

[10] ibid.

[11] Barnard, N., *Foods That Cause You To Lose Weight,* The Magni Group, McKinney, TX, 1992.

[12] Jordon, P., "Neuroendocrinology" American Fitness Magazine, Sherman Oaks, Ca., May/June 1988., p.38-40.

[13] Brody, J., *Jane Brody's Nutrition Book,* Bantam Books, NY, 1981. P. 317-320.

[14] Ibid., p. 319.

Chapter Three

The Dieting Dilemma

The result of conventional weight-loss-weight-regain diet cycles is inevitable. The more often you diet, the higher your body fat percentage can become.

Durk Pearson and Sandy Shaw
The Life Extension Weight-Loss Program[1]

Based on current nationwide statistics, Americans are gaining more weight than ever. Losing weight through on-and-off dieting has escalated. Current data actually shows that the number of individuals who are overweight outnumber the number of individuals maintaining normal weight. Because of these factors, many health experts contend that the long-standing practice of dieting in the traditional sense (calorie reduction) is outdated. This assumption is based on the fact that, on any given day, a large percentage of the American public is unsuccessfully dieting. An effective weight-and fat-loss program should include the following:

- Focus on reducing the size of fat cells;
- Curb and control appetite;
- Seek to maintain a high level of health;
- Provide a constant flow of balanced nutrition;
- Maintain existing energy levels;
- Be psychologically rewarding;
- Provide a means to maintain ideal weight;
- Encourage long-term habitual tendencies toward fat reduction and muscle-building;
- Encourage the elimination of poor dietary habits;
- Encourage changing sedentary lifestyles.

The reasons many traditional diets have a poor track record, is because they fail to adhere to these recommendations. However, the major problem with on-and-off dieting is that it causes the body to go into a survival mode. When you start reducing calorie intake, your body will store more fat than ever. In fact, once your body enters into survival mode, the metabolic rate (which determines how fast you burn calories) may remain depressed for up to a year after resuming a normal eating regime.

Measure your Body Fat

A recent survey conducted by the National Center for Health Statistics revealed that, for the first time ever, the number of people who are overweight in America is greater than the number of normal weight individuals. The results of this survey showed that 59 percent of American men and 49 percent of American women have "Body Mass Indexes" (Bemis) over 25. Current established guidelines for optimal health put proper Body Mass Indexes under 25.

The Body Mass Index, also known as the "Quetelet Index" is considered to be a much more reliable gauge relative to obesity. This assumption is based on the fact that traditional height and weight tables do not take into consideration how much of your total weight is actually body fat. To calculate your BMI, you would divide your total body weight (in kilograms) by your height (in centimeters). A body mass index over 25 indicates that you are overweight. Thirty and above indicates obesity.

Based on current standards, the body fat percentage for women is between 22 and 25%. Because of genetic makeup, women are naturally fatter than men. Women can classify themselves according to the following values as cited by Dr. William P. Marley, of the Human Performance Laboratory of the Holy Redeemer Hospital in Meadowbrook, PA:

The average acceptable range of body fat for women is:

Lean:	19.9% or less body fat
Average:	20% to 24.9% body fat
Overweight:	25% to 29.9% body fat
Obese:	30% or more body fat

The average acceptable range of body fat for men is:

Lean:	9.9% or less body fat
Average:	10% to 14.9% body fat
Overweight:	15% to 19.9% body fat
Obese:	20% or more body fat

Determining Your Body Mass Index

To determine your Body Mass Index, use the following formula: W/H^2. This formula is translated into the following equation: Weight (in kilograms)

_____

Height (in meters) x Height (in meters)

For example, a woman aged 24 weighs 46 Kg and is 1.57 meters tall:

$$46 / 1.57 \text{ x } 1.57 = 18.6$$

The index of 18.6 indicates that she is underweight.

To find out what your current body fat percentage is, please see figure 1.1 on the following page. To determine where you are in relationship to established body fat percent guideline, simply find your height and current weight measurements on the chart, intersect them and compare with the color key at the bottom of the chart.

Please note that the BMI is based on the metric system so the pounds are changed to kilograms and inches to centimeters. To change pounds to kilograms, divide your weight by 2.2, which equals 2.2 lbs. A meter is equal to 3.28 feet (which equals about 39 inches.)

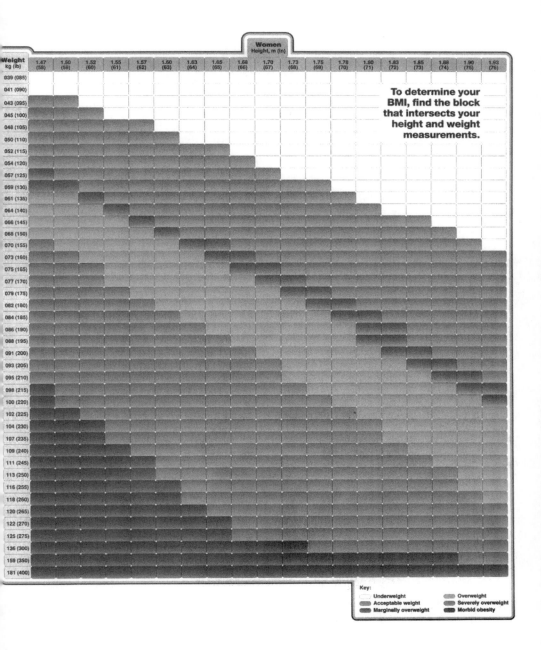

Figure 1.1
Source: David Sandler, "How Do You Measure Up?" Oxygen Magazine, Hollywood, FL, Jan/Feb 1999, p. 40.

Dr. Anthony Conte, M.D., a respected bariatric (obesity) physician and researcher, contends that obesity has ranked high on the list of national health problems. He went on to say that "today, more than a third of all adults in this country are obese (32 million women and 26 million men) and the numbers are rising, up 31% in the last ten years."[2]

Dr. Scott Connelly, M.D., a well-known physician who specializes in health, fitness and human nutrition, also maintains that Americans are getting fatter. Dr. Connelly of Met-Rx fame (a widely used food program for body builders) states that "despite all the diets, exercise programs, fat reduction creams, and liposuctions that have become commonplace in our society, Americans are still putting on the pounds."[3]

The above is astonishing when you consider the fact that on any given day, nearly half of all American women and a quarter of American men are dieting.

Every time the body is put on a very low calorie diet, it becomes more adept at existing on less food. According to Dr. Gillian Martlew, N.D., a member of the British Holistic Medical Association, when you go back to normal eating (whatever that may be for you) the body suddenly has more calories than it knows what to do with. The extra calories as perceived by your inborn genetic program, tells your body to store fat, hence the term "self defeating diet."[4] Dr. Robert Haas, a world renowned nutrition expert and author of *Eat Smart, Think Smart* and the best-selling book *Eat to Win*, cited a recent report that links yo-yo dieting to cancer. This study suggests that estrogen-like compounds stored in body fat, including pesticides from the environment, may cause breast, ovarian, endometrial (inner lining of uterus) and uterine cancer.[5]

According to Dr. Haas, the investigators of this study found that the major problem associated with the above findings correlate with the cycle of gaining weight as body fat and then losing it. During this cycle, two of the estrogen-mimicking pesticides, B-HCH (beta-hexachloro-cyclohexane) and "DDT" are stored in body fat and then released during weight loss when dieting. Dr. Haas maintains that when these powerful chemicals come in contact with reproductive organs, they can stimulate the unchecked cellular growth that leads to cancer.

Note: *DDT (Dichloro-Dphenyl-Trichloroethane) is a well-known pesticide, but it is also one of the most potent poisons known to humankind. Dr. Paul Herman Muller, the Swiss scientist who* *perfected DDT's use as an insecticide, was awarded the Nobel Prize in 1948. It was not until 1950 that a Congressional investigating committee revealed to the world that this agent could kill.[6] DDT is still used today and because we consume the foods it is sprayed on, it is estimated that most of us have two to seven parts per billion (PPB) of DDT in our blood system.[7]*

Set Point Theory

Current data suggest that the hypothalamus (the gland in the brain that controls weight) stimulates appetite just enough to help us maintain the level of body fat that the body has become accustomed to. Attempts to lower these levels (such as dieting) are often met with fierce resistance. Your fat cells are a major player in throwing up this wall of resistance. Scientists know that body fat is made up of millions of single fat cells all clamoring for their piece of pie. Most of these cells are acquired during early childhood, pre-adolescence and adolescence. Studies now confirm that these pockets of fat cells, if not already genetically programmed, can become part of your biological make-up for life.[8]

One of your best weapons against fat is muscle. Pound for pound, muscle keeps your metabolic rate on high, even when you sleep. When you diet, the body also fights to maintain precious muscle via the hypothalmus (your weight control center in the brain). Investigators believe that the body, to maintain its muscle mass at a constant level, seeks to have a set amount of amino acids (protein-building block) in the blood that is in proportion to your muscle mass. When this level drops below a certain point — which again signals the body's genetic survival mode — the hypothalamus signals you to eat to correct the situation. This phenomenon is referred to as the "set point theory."

This theory can be compared to your home's thermostat control, and your attempt at keeping your house at a certain temperature. Researchers have known for some time that laboratory animals will adjust food intake and physical activity to compensate for either too little available or too much food. When given small amounts of food, the animals are less active and when given too much, they exhibit much more activity. Investigators believe that the same kind of "set point" regulation exists in humans. This theory may explain why some people have difficulty in trying to lose as well as gain weight.

If you are seriously overweight, early efforts to lose weight can be very difficult. However, with persistent efforts body weight in time will change.

Although many diets initially cause a quick loss of weight, you must be aware that in many cases it is merely a rapid removal of water and vital electrolytes, not fat. Electrolytes are dissolved minerals that flow in the bloodstream and are responsible for conducting the "electrical impulses" which keep your heart and other vital organs working. Your life depends on maintaining this balance of water and electrolytes. This is why no matter what type of diet you select the focus, should be on fat loss versus loss of pounds. Overall health maintenance should be a main goal.

Scientists, however, remind us that even when pre-dispositioned with an excess of fat cells, although it may be difficult, a well-balanced meal plan and exercise program can bring you within normal weight ranges. In fact, according to Dr. Eric Peohlman, Ph.D., an obesity researcher at the University of Vermont College of Medicine in Burlington, about 30 to 40 percent of what we look like is regulated genetically. According to Dr. Peohlman, the rest is determined by lifestyle factors.

Persistence is the key. Persistence however, does not mean "constant dieting" but focuses on dynamic, well-balanced nutritional habits, movement and exercise. Based on the factors presented above, one could conclude that dieting will only make it more difficult to keep those unwanted pounds off.

If the body can sense something is wrong when calories are restricted, resulting in an increased fat storage, what is our alternative? According to Jamie Pope, M.S.R.D., author of the best-selling book the *T-Factor Fat Gram Counter, and The Last Five Pounds,* you must learn to eat, not diet. Jamie's term, eating refers to consuming four to six small meals a day versus one or two large meals. Ideally, these "mini meals" should be spread throughout the day. Eating smaller meals more frequently will help keep you metabolic rate on high, thus making it easier for you to get rid of unwanted pounds. By eating in this manner, your body will use what you eat for growth and repair of lean muscle, versus storing body fat. This is of vital importance if you are going to have any chance of reaching your goals. Knowing the correct amount of calories you need on a daily basis is a key factor to a sensible nutritional program.

It is very important that you understand you are in control. While genetics in some cases may play a role, you have the ability to modulate or control many of your body's own metabolic (fat-burning) processes. As cited by Dr. Barry Sears in his highly acclaimed book *Enter The Zone*, we should consider food as strong medicine, with the capability to manipulate our hormones and their ability, to help us lose and or cause us to gain weight. In other words, what, when and how much we eat, can determine if the body's fatburning capacity will increase or decrease.

Understanding Caloric Needs

Earlier in this chapter, we learned about the set point theory, which says that our body seeks to maintain a certain weight level based on individual biochemical or biological makeup. Current thinking suggests that while calorie intake is an important variable (motivating factor) in the weight loss equation, determining just how many calories you need to shed pounds can be built right into the equation. To do this, you will need the following:

- your basal metabolic rate;
- the number of calories you expend during activities;
- your total daily energy needs.

Basal metabolic rate (BMR) is concerned with the number of calories you need to maintain normal everyday bodily processes (even sleeping) when your body is at rest. Your activity and energy calorie needs revolve around the calories you expend throughout the day.

Think of metabolism as the furnace that burns the food you eat and transforms it into the energy your body requires to function. Your individual "metabolic rate" is the speed at which this takes place.

Factors that Affect Metabolism

In addition to the above, there are three main factors that determine or manipulate your metabolic rate.

- Your RMR: RMR stands for "resting metabolic rate." This factor is concerned with the energy required to sustain your body functions on a day-to-day basis. Bodily functions pertain to the heart pumping, respiration and cell functions.
  Note: This expenditure of energy has to be maintained from 60 to 75 percent of the calories you consume each day.

- <u>Your Activity</u>: The energy you use or need to keep up with your daily activities, such as housework, going swimming, walking and/or exercising.

- <u>What You Eat</u>: This third factor, often overlooked and/or not given much consideration by many, is called the metabolic pathways with each step started by a specific enzyme.[9]

Determining Metabolic Capacity

As stated, metabolism is concerned with how effectively your body is carrying out its vital chemical processes. According to Brenda Garrison, R.D., of the Cooper Wellness Program in Dallas, TX, there are several ways to test human metabolic activity. Through the use of a device that measures oxygen intake and carbon dioxide loss (a metabolic by-product), you can determine how well you are expending energy.[10] Although tests may reveal that you are expending energy at established normal rates, you can inadvertently slow down metabolic activity via poor and inappropriate calorie and food choices. Dr. Martin Katahan, former Director of The Weight Management Program at Vanderbilt University in Nashville, TN puts the above assumptions into proper perspective with the following comments. "You can be born with a fast metabolism, although your eating habits and lifestyle can change a perfectly normal or thin metabolism into a fat one."[11]

To ensure you are giving your body the correct ratios of the raw material (food) it needs for peak metabolic activity, it is important to know just how many calories you as an individual need to sustain your metabolic processes. This will require some caloric awareness on your part to ensure that you stay within accepted parameters, in reference to food calories needed, energy expenditures, and the relationship to weight and fat loss management. By following the guidelines of the following worksheet, you will be able to establish your baseline of calories needed to:
- maintain your present weight;
- stimulate metabolic activity to burn body fat;
- maintain energy levels for physical activity; and
- maintain internal life processes.

How to Determine Individual Calorie Requirements

Calorie awareness is important for people who are trying to lose weight. But before you can determine the number of calories you should have daily in order to shed excess pounds, you must figure out how many you need to maintain your present weight. This depends on two elements: your basal metabolic rate and the number of calories you expend during daily activities.

Your basal metabolic rate (BMR) refers to the number of calories you require to maintain normal bodily processes when your body is at rest. You can determine your BMR by following the simple steps below:

Example for a 150-pound woman:

Step #1:   Change pounds to kilograms (divide your weight by 2.2) ex:150 lb. ÷ 2.2 lbs. / kg =68kg

Step #2:   Multiply weight in kilograms by the BMR factor. For men the factor is 1.0 and for women it is 0.9 ex: 68 kg x 0.9 cal / kg / hr = 61 cal / hr.

Step #3   Multiply the calories used in one hour by the 24 (hours in a day).

One thousand four hundred sixty four (1464) represents the BMR, which is the number of calories that are needed to maintain life processes: respiration, heartbeat, maintenance of body temperature, and other essential functions.

As previously discussed, many of us do not take into consideration what we eat and its effect on metabolic activity. Understanding the concept of calorie intake is vital in assisting you with reaching and maintaining your weight and fat loss goals.

In the next chapter, we will take a look at our dependence on drugs versus our reliance on adhering to some basic principles that increase our potential to remain healthy and within normal established weight and body fat guidelines. We will also take a look at the legalities of manufacturing drugs, the cost, and more importantly, an industry intent of ensuring that you the consumer, continue to practice treatment versus prevention.

---

[1] Pearson, D., Shaw, S., *The Life Extension Weight Loss Program*, Doubleday and Co., Garden City, NY, 1986.

[2] Conte, A. A., "A Non-prescription Alternative in Weight Reduction Therapy," The Bariatrician, Summer, 1993, p. 17-19.

[3] Connelly S., *America, Land of the Fat*, The Connelly Report, Irvine CA., No. 12, Dec. 1994.

[4] Martlew, G., Electrolytes: *The Spark of Life*, Natures Publishing, LTD., Murdock, FL, 1994, p. 50.

[5] Haas, R., "Yo Yo Dieting Linked To Cancer," All Natural Muscular Development, Ronkokoman, NY, Sept. 1997, p. 168.

[6] Null, G., Null, S., *How To Get Rid of The Poisons In Your Body,* Prentice Hall Press, NY, 1977, p 168-169.

[7] Crosby, S.W., "How To Thrive On An Ailing Planet," Ms Fitness Magazine, Corona CA, Summer 1997, p.76-78.

[8] Morgan, B.L.G., Morgan R. *Hormones: How They Affect Behavior, Metabolism, Growth, Development and Relationships,* The Body Press, Los Angles CA, 1989.

[9] Campbell, R. A., *Biology, 3rd Edition,* Benjamin Cummings, Redwood City, CA, 1993.

[10] Penn, F., "Cheat and Beat Your Metabolism," Fitness Magazine, New York, NY, May, 1997, p. 80-85.

[11] Katahn, M., *Beyond Diet, The 28 Day Metobolic Breakthrough Plan,* Berkley Books, NY, 1984, p. 15.

Chapter Four

Dying To Be Thin

The health benefits of Fenfluramine and dexfenflu-ramine outweigh the risk 20 to 1. It is estimated that 280 lives would be saved per million users of fen-phen compared to an estimated 14 deaths. An additional 400 non-fatal heart attacks and strokes would also be prevented.

Mason and Faich
Pharmacotherapy for Obesity, New England Journal of Medicine, 1996 [1]

Are You Confused Yet?

When you read the opening remarks in regards to the life-saving capabilities of the once-infamous diet drug called fen-phen, and compare them to the statements made by several prominent health care officials in the prologue of this report concerning its lethal capabilities, which door would you have chosen? Door number one reveals research that shows serious long-term health complications up to and including death by using this diet drug. Door number two cites a report in the prestigious New England Journal of Medicine[2] that claims this drug and others like it were the most viable option in preventing any further complications to existing health problems associated with obesity, including saving your life.

Many individuals make monumental decisions that may have far-reaching implications for the future of their overall health. When comments are made and appear in such prestigious publications like the New England Journal of Medicine, it is difficult not to follow the advice of these prominent researchers. For many Americans who chose the fen-phen combo to help support their weight loss efforts, many have fallen prey to the negative and/or deadly consequences behind door number one.

Take for example the case of former Philadelphia Phillies professional baseball player Randy Ready. Ready won a $24.7 million judgment in 1990 against a physician who prescribed Phenten-nine Chloride for his wife. Dorene Ready should not have been placed on the drug as she did not fit the established guidelines proposed by the FDA which states that, to be considered a candidate for the drug's use, you must be 20 percent overweight. As a result of the drug, she became "crippled" and "speechless" and unable to care for herself due to brain damage suffered in a massive cardiac arrest (heart attack).[3]

Consider also the circumstances surrounding the death of Josie Freeman, a housewife, who was prescribed the fen-phen combo apparently over the phone.[4] In February 1996, Josie developed a cough, which lingered through that same summer until late October. She became breathless just by walking from the bed to the bathroom, and was unable to work. On November 20th, 1996, her lungs finally gave out on her as a result of pulmonary hypertension, a rare disorder in which blood pressure increases in the lungs causing congestive heart failure.[5] During the initial frenzy and reported cases of quick and, in some cases, dramatic weight loss, Redux (fen-phen) had been prescribed at a rate of about 65,000 new prescriptions per week. Launched in June of 1996 as a new miracle diet pill, fen-phen lost much of its steam in the early part of 1997 as reports began pouring in concerning many negative side effects of this drug. These included mood swings, severe depression, unexplained fatigue, headaches, vivid dreams, lung disease, drowsiness, possible brain damage, lapses of unconsciousness and even death.

With all the uncertainty surrounding the safety of this new diet drug, widespread abuse continued. On July 4, 1997, on the award-winning TV show 20/20, it was reported that several people had died of or had contracted the fatal lung disease Primary Pulmonary Hypertension. In addition to the above, there were conflicting reports concerning the drug's ability to cause irreversible brain damage, known medically as neurotoxicity. As stated by Dr. Lewis Ruben, a top U. S. expert on primary pulmonary hypertension (PPH) on the 20/20 program, the question was asked, "How many young women need develop a fatal disease from taking this drug, before we start asking questions?"

Furthermore, Lynn McAfee, the Director of the Medical Education Project for the Council on Size and Weight Discrimination, posed the following questions. "Are we changing from generations of being labeled as 'morally inferior' because of what is perceived to be a lack of willpower; and, if that is changing, as being fat is increasingly being seen as a disease, are those who are obese in danger of being labeled biologically inferior?"[6]

Despite all the excitement concerning this new era and the problems cited with the use of these diet drugs, mass mania and misapplication of the drugs was still going strong. Even more alarming is that no one knows for sure what the long-term effects will be. In fact, according to the FDA, the safety and effectiveness of Redux beyond one year had not been determined.[7]

According to University Medical Research Publishers in their report, *Amazing Medicines the Drug Companies Don't Want You To Discover,*[8] there are interesting facts about the relationship between drug companies and the Food and Drug Administration (FDA). These researchers contend that the FDA, in some cases, play a role in the widespread greed that exists within this industry. Dr. Gillian Martlew, N.D., maintains that there are powerful influences that determine our health and care.[9] She argues vehemently that drug and chemical companies have billions of dollars invested in their products and high sums in money are spent on research. According to previous reports in *Chemical World*, a magazine that serves the pharmaceutical industry, the pharmaceutical business is one of the most profitable in the world. In fact, as stated by Donald Drake and Marian Uhlman, "It doesn't matter if the economy is flourishing or stagnant, if the jobless rates are high or low, or if America is at war or peace, the pharmaceutical industry rakes in cash. No other legal business consistently makes as large a profit."[10]

This is in part due to the fact that pharmaceutical companies are awarded monopolies on a newly patented drug for 17 years and they can charge any price they wish. No person, company, or other drug manufacturer can create a generic copy of a newly approved drug for that same 17-year period. Drake and Uhlman, however, argue in their report that drug companies have circumvented every governmental effort to bring prices under control, and are granted monopoly markets along with the opportunity to profit from research findings by government and academic scientists. The most insidious observations the reports bring to light is the fact that these giants often put high price tags on drugs that have been developed via taxpayer funded research. In many cases, the public is getting a double whammy financially in reference to drug use.

This point is also made by Dr. Andrew Weil, M.D., who is both a medical researcher and a world-renowned physician and medical botanist. Dr. Weil states, "in this country, the creation of new drugs in laboratories has shifted from university to industry, with large pharmaceutical companies vying with one another to come up with marketable drugs that are innovative, with greater potency; strength and rapidity of action remain the qualities sought, and increasingly, novelty has become a desired characteristic."[11]

Dr. Weil also makes note of the fact that in some cases drug companies may remarket drugs for different purposes. In many instances, FDA approval costs a minimum of ten million dollars. In an article titled "Brave New Drug World,"[12] researchers contend that drugs which already have been approved to treat obesity, will most likely be repackaged and marketed as anorexiants (appetite suppressants).

A commentary from *Allure Magazine*,[13] reports that a division of Eli Lilly intends to redistribute Prozac, (the widely prescribed anti-depressant drug) as a diet aid. Named Lovan, this drug will be remarketed due to the fact that Prozac users have reported an average weight loss of two to three pounds. This practice is very dangerous, as cited by Dr. Martlew, whom I spoke of earlier.

It costs an average of 231 million plus dollars to bring a new prescription drug to the marketplace in the United States. Pharmaceutical companies are cashing in on the quest to be thin at any cost. Traditionally, drug manufacturers target physicians. However, this trend is changing. Because of technological advances, drug companies have shifted their focus to the buying public. Pharmaceutical companies know that while the doctor writes the prescription, it is the patient who guides the pen. An estimated one-third of all new prescriptions are now written at the request of the patient[14].

While drug companies today can actually create public demand via the media, their primary customer remains your physician. In a recent study[15] done by David Phillips of the University of California at San Diego, it was revealed that many medical doctors initially receive their knowledge about new drugs through the newspapers. Only after they read recent news stories do they decide which products are worth the time to review the scientific literature on them.

The above sentiments also were expressed by Donald Drake and Marian Uhlman of The Philadelphia Inquirer Newspaper. In their award-winning investigative report, they revealed that when physicians write prescriptions, most patients assume their doctors choose a drug based on scientific research, knowledge, and an educational level well beyond their own. However, you may be shocked to find out this is far from the truth. These reporters state, "Doctors are taught only general principles of pharmacology in medical school classes. Their practical knowledge comes from on-the-job training where treatment choices often are influenced by which drugs are on their medical center's formulary. That in turn, is influenced by the marketing skills of drug companies."[16]

Moreover, several consumer groups have recently criticized drug companies who pressure doctors. Ohio Senator Howard Metzenbaum, who has served as Chairman of the Consumer Federation of America, calls their actions "the best kept secret in health care."[17] Metzenbaum contends that [drug companies] have taken control over the kinds of prescriptions available to patients within our medical system. Consumer groups maintain that pharmaceutical giants are buying "drug benefit management" companies (PBMs) to gain control and monopolize which prescription drugs, listed as formularies, are allowed by health insurance plans. Furthermore, under oath at several recent Congressional Hearings, medical experts and several industry analysts cited numerous negative measures used by the drug industry to deceive the public via media outlets. As reported in Consumer Reports Magazine,[18] drug companies contract doctors to act as paid spokespersons. They are passed off as independent unbiased experts and in many cases, although touted as breakthroughs, the drugs they promote offer little advantage over older formulations. To make matters worse, in some cases, unapproved and even untested uses of drugs are broadcast via press conferences and press releases.[19]

A recent survey[20] conducted by the National Center for Health Statistics has revealed that for the first time ever, the number of people that are overweight in America, exceed the number of people carrying a normal weight. The above survey, which was done from 1991 to 1994 on 30,000 people, showed that 59 percent of American men and 49 percent of American women have Body Mass Indexes (BMIs) over 25. According to current established guidelines for optimal health, body mass indexes should be under 25.

How important is this fact? Consider the data as reported in a recent Ni Hanes III study,[21] conducted by the National Institute of Health in Maryland. This study reveals that of the individuals with Body Mass Indexes (BMI's) over 25 in many cases 70 percent have type 2 diabetes, 56 percent have hypertension, and 47 percent have high cholesterol.

Like a scene from a horror movie, Americans are dying slowly and silently. We are perpetuating our own genocide. Diabetes is 2.57 times more prevalent in overweight persons than in normal weight persons. Current data shows that Americans have the highest incidence of death from diabetes over any nation in the world. Also, death rates from cancer and heart disease are greater in those who are overweight. Degenerative circulatory conditions in males who are 5 to 15 percent overweight are 44 percent higher than in men of normal weight, and twice as high in individuals 15 to 25 percent overweight. As suggested by Dr. H. Curtis Wood, Jr., M.D.,[22] these figures have great significance since cardiovascular disease continues to kill more Americans than all other causes of death, and more "fat" people die of various conditions related to diet and sedentary lifestyles than normal weight persons.

How Fat Are You?

Health experts claim that fat tissue accounts for a high percentage of total body weight. Today, this barometer is used as an indication of the possible onset of various disease states. Most people fail to realize the cycle of consuming excess calories and its role in storing fat for future use. If not utilized, storage continues until those fat cells begin to split into two fat cells. Once you have this new fat cell, you have it for life![23]

There are ways you can naturally reduce the size of these fat cells, which we will cover in a subsequent chapter. However, a strong, determined, consistent and committed effort will be needed to accomplish this. Let's repeat the above message again loud and clear!

> *If extra calories are not needed, they are stored as body fat in fat cells. Once these cells become full, they begin to split in two and forms a new fat cell. Once you have this new fat cell you have it for life!*

On the television show 20/20, Dr. Ruben asked as a society how many people have to die before we admit that there are serious complications associated with the use of fen-phen. Many people had to die and develop heart valve abnormalities before diet drugs were banned on September 15, 1997 by the FDA. Heart valve problems were reported in 32 percent of diet drug users. To date, cardiologist Dr. Heidi Connolly of the prestigious Mayo Clinic, claims that there are now 100 known cases of people with this condition related to diet drugs. Ongoing studies question whether or not the problems related to PPH (Primary Pulmonary Hypertension) go away when the patient stops taking the diet drug or do the problems continue throughout life and for how long. One fact that is known, according to medical researchers, is that 50 percent of those individuals who contract PPH will eventually die prematurely. For many persons who contracted this disorder, finding the answers to these questions will become paramount as the nightmare unfolds.

Take, for example, the probability of Ms. Rose Jones[24] of Santa Cruz, California, a 45-year-old computer consultant, who had to quit her job after several years of being on fen-phen. Although she received a substantial settlement through a lawsuit, she is being kept alive with a medication fed intravenously through a pump she must wear all the time.

To complicate matters more, our society has become enormously dependent on the doctor-patient relationship. This encourages people to shift responsibility to the physician for maintaining health and preventing serious related problems. Dr. Donald M. Vickery, reminds us that in the early 1970s death rates began to decline at a significant rate. He points out this decline correlates with reduced use of tobacco, less saturated fats and cholesterol in the diet, and more importantly increased exercise among adults. He also argues vehemently that the "miracles of modern medicine" had little to do with the long-term declines in the death rate. Dr. Vickery insists that we appear to be in an era where life-styles rather than medicine will be the dominant factor deciding further gains in health.[25]

Dr. John W. Farquhar, M.D., Director of the renowned Stanford Center for Research in Disease Prevention, and Professor of Medicine at Stanford University, cautions us about the daily lifestyle choices that we make as a result of powerful complex influences within our culture. Dr. Farquhar challenges each and every one of us not to fall prey to missed opportunities for illness prevention. He maintains that, "we need to stop making excuses and need to stop expecting a cure-all somewhere out there to compensate for unhealthy living patterns."[26]

As a society, it seems we have lost our way, and have become mirrored images of the technology that surrounds us. We seek quick fixes, placing profits and economic gain before the safety and welfare of ourselves. This point so adamantly portrayed by Dr. Martlew, seems to imply that you the individual may have little recourse to protect and preserve your health potential. This is quite to the contrary. You do have some clear cut viable options to this new era of potentially lethal diet drugs.

A new study conducted by the Health Policy Institute at the Medical College of Wisconsin in Milwaukee, estimates that by the year 2010, the supply of alternative medical clinics will increase by 124 percent.[27] Furthermore, responding to consumer demand, the National Institute of Health, Office of Alternative Medicine (established in 1992) has allocated millions of dollars in grants for research on how diets, plants, supplements and exercise counteract or help alleviate problems related to obesity. In fact dollars allocated for research on dietary supplements and the efficacy of alternative medical protocols have skyrocketed over the last few years. As recently as March 2001, the United States Congress allocated a 30-percent increase (from 50to 89 million dollars) in the budget for the National Institutes of Health's (NIH) National Center for Complementary and Alternative Medicine. Additionally, Congress increased the NIH's office of Dietary Supplements Budget to 10 million dollars.

A silent but active revolution is at work amidst all this confusion surrounding diet drugs. There are presently many viable alternatives. Later in this book, we will review current research concerning many of the most popular natural fatburning supplements. However, in the next chapter, we will review some past and present diet drugs and examine the critical differences synthetic medications have on human physiology versus their natural counterparts.

---

[1] Mason, J.E., Faich, G.A., "Pharmacotherapy For Obesity – Do The Benefits Outweigh the Risk?" New England Journal of Medicine 8:29:1996, 335 (9) 659-60.

[2] ibid.

[3] Knox, A. "Relying On Pills To Pull The Weight, Phila. Inquirer, Phila. PA, 1997.

[4] Levine, H., "Fen-phen Killed My Wife," Cosmopolitan Magazine, December, 1997, p.196-199.

[5] ibid. p. 198.

[6] McAfee, L., Redux: "Is Weight Loss Worth It?" Labyrinth, The Philadelphia Women's Newspaper, Westbury Publishing Inc., Phila. PA: Vol. 15, No 1 1997.

[7] Fox, M., Stanten, M., "Diet Pills Boom or Bust?" Prevention Magazine, Emmas PA., April, 1997, Vol. 49, No. 4, p. 92-95.

[8] Kugler, H.J., Amazing Medicines Drug Companies, Don't Want You To Discover, Tempe AZ: University Medical Research Publishers, 1999.

[9] Martlew, G., Electrolytes: The Spark of Life, Natures Publishing, LTD., Murdock, FL 1994.

[10] Drake, D., Uhlman, M., *Making Medicine Making Money,* Andrew and McMeel Publishing, NY, 1993.

[11] Weil A., *Health and Healing,* Houghton-Mifflin Company, Boston, MA,1995.

[12] Clive, T., "Brave New Drug World, Can Phen-Fen Really Make You Thinner?" Iron Man magazine, Oxnard, CA Feb., 1997, p. 102-103.

[13] Ibid.

[14] Landau, I (ED.), "Miracle Drugs or Media Drugs", Consumer Reports, Yonkers NY., March 1992, p. 142-146.

[15] Ibid.

[16] Drake, D., Uhlman. M., *Making Medicine Making Money,* Andrew & McMeel Publishing, NY, 1993.

[17] DNE Pharmaceuticals, "Consumer Groups Criticize Drug Companies", Diet, Nutrition and Energy News, Bloomingdale, NJ, Oct./Nov., 1997, p.9.

[18] Landau, I (ED.), "Miracle Drugs or Media Drugs", Consumer Reports, Yonkers NY., March 1992, p. 142-146.

[19] Ibid.

[20] Fahey, T.D., "Obesity In America: Body Mass Index and Obesity", All Natural Muscular Development Vol. 32, No. 2 Feb 2000, Rokonkoma, NY, p.62-63.

[21] National Institute Health (NIH) "Methods for voluntary weight loss and control, NIH Technology Assessment Conference Panel", Annals of Internal Medicine, 1165: June 1992, 942-949.

[22] Wood, H.C., *Overfed But Undernourished,* Exposition Press, Inc., NY, 1959.

[23] Pike, R., Brown, M. L., *Nutrition: An Integrated Approach,* , MacMillan Publishing, New York, NY, 1984, p. 177

[24] Johannes, L., Schmitt, R.B., "Lawyers Prepare for Deluge of Diet Drug Suits", Wall Street Journal, Sept. 17, 1997, Section B, P, and P.10.

[25] Vickery, D.M., *Life Plan For Your Health*, Addison Wesley, Reading MA,1978, p.7-8.

[26] Farguar, J.W., "The American Way of Life Need Not Be Hazardous To Your Health," Stanford Alumni Assoc., Stanford, CA, 1987.

[27] "The Politics of Medicine 31% of Americans left out in the cold, Despite $1 trillion for U.S. Healthcare", Alternative Medicine Digest,Tiburon, CA. Issue 16: 82-83.

Chapter Five

Winning without Diet Drugs

People who say it cannot be done should not interfere or interrupt those who are doing it.

The Silver Lining[1]

A recent study, which appeared in the New England Journal of Medicine, revealed that thirty-four percent of Americans now use some form of complementary or alternative health care service. During this survey period, the dollars spent on these unconventional therapies totaled over 13.7 billion dollars.[2] Being unfamiliar with alternative healthcare, or lacking knowledge about products and their efficacy may prevent many consumers from seeking advice outside of their normal channels (medical doctors). This however is changing rapidly.

The Politics of Manufacturing Drugs

It takes millions of dollars and many years of research to bring a drug to the marketplace. Once approved for human use and patented, drug companies have the exclusive right to market and sell the said product for a seventeen-year period. This is not the case with a natural substance. No one can patent lecithin, CoQ10, cayenne, chromium, water (H_2o), pyruvate, L-carnitine, grapefruit extract or various kinds of plant-derived products. Because of the above factors, medical doctors and pharmaceutical companies have had little interest in marketing these products.

On average, as cited by Donald Drake and Marian Uhlman, it costs drug companies over 200 million dollars to bring a drug to the marketplace. They are unwilling to make this kind of investment in a natural product which they cannot patent, market and set prices for. According to Drake and Ulman, it is a 55 billion dollar a year industry that is at stake. These authors state that drug companies spend about 10 billion dollars a year on advertising, three billion on sales representatives, and at least 500 million dollars on ads in top medical journals. Their goal is to market to medical doctors and prescribing physicians. In financial terms, drug companies spend about $13,000 marketing to each doctor. This ultimately influences the type of medical treatment a patient receives and the drug prescribed.

Drake and Uhlman also make note of a statement made by Harvard Medical School professor Terry Avorn who believed that the best way to control rising drug prices is by providing physicians with accurate and timely information on the best and most cost-effective drugs. However, he cautions that if we as a society leave it up to the manufacturers of drugs to be the only purveyors of information, then we shouldn't expect them to do anything but try to increase sales.[3]

It is estimated that weight loss sales in the United States will reach 34.6 billion dollars in the year 2002.[4] However, as cited earlier, there is a changing trend among Americans who are seeking ways to lose unwanted fat and pounds safely and effectively without compromising their health. Consumers are exploring natural products and are reaping great success. According to Catherine Valenti of ABCNEWS.com, sales of healthier meal replacements, natural fatburners, and appetite suppressants are expected to reach 1.7 billion dollars by the end of 2001. These estimates represent almost a 15 percent increase from 1999.[5]

This trend has been steadily gaining momentum over the last decade. A 1990 consumer survey by *Whole Foods Magazine* revealed that 11 percent of individuals who purchased products from natural health stores use a natural diet or fatburning aid.[6] Today those percentages have skyrocketed, as consumers want safer and more cost-effective ways to reach their weight and fat-loss goals. Marketdata Enterprises, Inc., with more than 37,000 research publications from over 350 leading consulting and advisory firms, confirmed that sales of non-prescription diet aids and supplements were up 90 percent.[7]

Recently, nationally syndicated shows such as 20/20 and others have begun to air reports of the benefits of natural substances. For example, they compared St. John's Wort, a natural alternative to Prozac for fighting depression. The media has given coverage to the fat-fighting ability of natural products like Xenadrine rfa-1 and Metabolife 356. Xenadrine rfa-1 is being touted as a leading natural fatburning supplement, while Metabolife sales have reached ten million dollars. Why all the hoopla? People using these products and many of the alternative diet regimes have had great success. As an added benefit, you do not have to jeopardize your health or your life. Dr. David Levitsky, PH.D. Professor of Nutrition and Psychology at

Cornell University says, "Weight loss with Fenfluramine and other diet drugs average less than 20 pounds in a year of dieting as compared to more than 14 pounds lost per year when subjects take placebos."[8] Replacements for the Fen-phen combo are on the horizon. It is this author's contention that you must resist the quick fix approach and the risk to your health

In some laboratory or manufacturing plants, new versions of diet drugs are poised to flood the marketplace. The incentive for financial gain from diet drugs more than compensates for research dollars spent. As history has already indicated, profit incentives may outweigh the potential associated health risk to the consumer. However, Dr. Sherry A. Rodgers, M.D., contends, "there is a nutrient or nutrient for nearly every drug that accomplishes the same function in the body."[9]

Dr. Rogers also says, "the only difference is when the problem has been attacked from a biochemical/nutritional basis, the problem is usually solved or cured." This statement reminds us that food, when used properly, is your best medicine as it assists the body in its healing and recouperative powers as well as its inborn fatburning capabilities.

There is definitely a correlation between what you eat and the body's ability to metabolize (break down) the food. In his book *Fit For Life,* well-known nutritionist, Harvey Diamond reminds us of the "Theory of Metabolic Capacity."[10] It explains how toxemia, which develops due to the improper breakdown of food, directly contributes to our inability to control weight. This theory, relating food to our metabolic (fatburning) capacity can be explained by examining your diet.

Let's say your eating regime is composed primarily of highly processed foods, red meats, and a diet devoid of fiber and enzymes. Because these particular foods are more difficult for the body to metabolize, the "unprocessed" food accumulates faster than the body can get rid of it. Mr. Diamond says, "If you have any kind of weight problem, this is what your body has to deal with. If you build up more toxic waste every day than what is eliminated, it has to be stored somewhere. Your body, ever attempting to protect itself and maintain its integrity, tends not to store this waste in or near the vital organs."[11]

An analogy compares our digestive system to a drainpipe in your home that seems to be forever clogging up. Imagine pouring the scraps of food you have decided not to eat down that sink.

Without a garbage disposal, the pipe will remain sluggish with each and every scrap of food you put down there. The scrapes of food cannot be processed, so they continue to accumulate until the sink becomes completely clogged.

The body uses fatty tissue and muscle as dumpsites, resulting in unsightly cellulite indentations in the thighs, buttocks, around the midsection, and the upper arms. If left unchecked, this process may lead to obesity, as well as general discomfort and lethargy. This is due to the fact that the body expends an enormous amount of its energy pool trying to get rid of this accumulated waste. But you can take control of this situation. You have the capability to end this vicious cycle of continuous weight gain — *right now*!

In reducing or eliminating the risk factors and other problems associated with obesity, patience and persistence are keys. They are your allies. Use them judiciously and you can begin to reduce the accumulated waste by-products.

Restoring metobolic (fatburning) capacity with food

In order to shed those pounds, you must learn how to eat — not diet. You can turn this negative spiral around safely and effectively by making a few changes in types of foods you are eating. In a few short weeks, you can actually switch your metabolic capacity from "Park" to "Turbo Drive". Yes, there are foods that have the ability to act as natural fatburners. They actually fuel your innate metabolic system and help to keep this natural cycle in high gear. In essence, you can shift your own metabolic cycle from what obesity researchers classify individuals as a slow-burner to a fast-burner.

As stated before, the key is patient and persistence. Do not expect to lose fifty pounds overnight. Losing one pound per week is safer, and in the long run a much healthier solution. To be effective, we must switch the throttles of our metabolic or fatburning capacity. By giving attention to your goal and not your present weight, you may find it easier to avoid the temptation of dangerous diet drugs. You will be less pressured, more relaxed about the program, and may easily rebuild your self-confidence, self-esteem and self-control.

The Plan

To begin I want you to start by playing the exchange game. Right now I want you to slowly reduce or eliminate your intake of the following foods:

- white bread
- white rice
- white flour
- potato chips
- soda pop
- refined cereal
- salt
- eggs
- bacon
- milk
- butter
- cream
- hot dogs
- cold cuts

- mashed potato
- red organ meats
- ice cream
- canned fruits and vegetables
- pies, cakes, cookies
- frozen fruits and vegetables
- candy
- alcohol
- fast foods
- sugar (white)
- sausage
- potato chips
- fruits in heavy syrup
- pork sausages

I know you are asking if there is anything left to eat. Most of these foods are the staple of the American diet. Consider the selections of *101 Fatburning Foods* listed on the next page. They actually assist the body in breaking down and utilizing fat as a fuel, and these foods may actually contain considerably less fat themselves. They also help the body to stabilize blood sugar levels, which contributes to the process of maintaining more lean muscle. Finally, many of these foods also have a high water content. Why is this important? We are predominately made up of water. It is water that transports the nutrients in foods to your cells. Water also is vital to your body's ability to remove toxic waste by-products. You will find that many of these fatburning foods are common to your present diet — we just do not consume enough of them!

You did not gain those extra pounds overnight. They will not go away overnight. Have patience! In the absence of any congenital defects or metabolic disorders such as thyroid dysfunction, you can reach your goal. Even when faced with some minor metabolic disorders, you can still win.

101 Fatburning Foods

Consume More of These Fatburning Foods

1. fresh fruits
2. fresh vegetables
3. sherbet
4. yogurt
5. soy products
6. olive oil
7. flax seed oil
8. whole wheat, rye flour
9. unpasteurized dairy products
10. sugar substitutes
11. whole wheat pasta
12. chicken (white meat) with skin removed
13. tuna
14. apples
15. bananas
16. popcorn (air popped no butter)
17. fructose
18. apple cider vinegar (raw)
19. low-fat snacks (all kinds)
20. lentils
21. broccoli
22. carrots
23. veggie hamburgers, hot dogs
24. oatmeal
25. dark green leafy vegetables
26. whole wheat spaghetti
27. grapefruit
28. sunflower seeds
29. wheat germ
30. nutritional yeast
31. brussel sprouts
32 collard greens
65. yams
66. rye bread

33. unsweetened fruit juice
34. raw nuts and seeds
35. tofu
36. melon
37. whole grain bread
38. brown rice
39. bulgur and cracked wheat
40. goat's milk
41. legumes (ex: lentils, navy beans)
42. oat bran
43. cottage cheese
44. lean cuts of meats (about 4oz. per meal)
45. corn
46. raisins
47. rice cakes
48. egg substitutes (fat free)
49. dates, apricots
50. tomatoes
51. non-alcoholic beverages
52. peas
53. canola oil
54. soy mayonnaise
55. strawberries
56. prunes
57. cabbage
58. scallops
59. low-fat dairy products
60. flavored water (no sugar)
61. pinto beans
62. celery stalks
63. baked chicken
64. green beans
83. cherries
84. bacon bits (non-fat)

67. turkey	85. buckwheat
68. salmon	86. oat flour
69. swordfish	87. rice (basmati, wild)
70. halibut	88. egg whites
71. water (eight glasses daily)	89. pumpkin
72. herb dressings	90. lettuce
73. amaranth	91. soybeans
74. artichoke pasta	92. black-eyed peas
75. rice bran	93. peanut butter (sparingly)
76. cantaloupe	94. cheese (low-fat)
77. honeydew	95. puffed rice
78. tangerines	96. cucumbers
79. garlic	97. red onions
80. steamed potatoes	98. kasha
81. red potatoes	99. pineapple
82. whole grain noodles	100. blueberries
	101. beets

Taking The First Step

The first step in the weight-loss process is actually the easiest. You will have total control. Once you begin to make gradual subtle changes — what, when and how much you eat — the other aspects concerning fatburning supplements and exercise will easily and effectively shift your natural metabolic (fatburning) cycle into high gear.

While this list above represents only the tip of the iceberg concerning your choices of fatburning foods, there are literally thousands of combinations and delicious recipes at your disposal. To assist you in broadening your choices and knowledge of the body's metabolic capacity, use the list of suggested reading below.

- *Eating Thin For Life*, Anne M. Fletcher; Chapters Publishing
- *Fit For Life*, Harvey and Marilyn Diamond, Warner Books
- *Genetic Nutrition*, Artemis P. Simopoulos, Victor Herbert, Beverly Jacobson, MacMillan Publishing
- *Lean Bodies*, Cliff Sheats and Maggie Greenwood-Robinson, Warner Books
- *Maximum Metabolism*, Robert M. Giller, and Kathy Matthews, G.P. Putnam Sons
- *Metabolics: Putting Your Food Energy To Work*, Lawrence Lamb, Harper and Row

- *Metabolize: The Personalized Program For Weight Loss*, Kenneth Baum; G.P. Putnam and Sons
- *Power Eating*, Susan M. Kleiner, Human Kinetics
- *The Underburner's Diet*, Barbara Edelstein, MacMillan Publishing Co.
- *Weight Watchers 15-Minute Cookbook*, Deborah Garrison Lowery, (Editor), Oxmor House Inc.

For now I want to encourage you to eat by the creed above. Utilize more enzyme-packed and fiber-rich fatburning foods. Leave the scientific jargon at the door, and focus on giving your body more of what it needs and less of what it doesn't. Consume a variety of foods every day, but eat in moderation. This way you will be assured of getting adequate intake proteins and carbohydrates.

Dr. Susan Kleiner, an authority on eating for strength and who has served as the nutritional consultant to the Cleveland Cavaliers of the NBA, states that carbohydrates are the real force behind muscle building and fatburning. She reminds us that the body burns fat for energy that takes place inside the cells. She asks us to think of fat as a log in the fireplace waiting to be ignited. According to Dr. Kleiner, carbohydrate is the match that ignites fat at the cellular level.[12] Another benefit, especially the consumption of complex carbohydrates versus simple carbohydrates, is that complex carbohydrates encourage the production of serotonin in the brain.[13] Serotonin is what the diet drug fen-phen was suppose to elevate as it increases feelings of calmness, improves sleep patterns and actually reduces cravings for carbohydrates. Focus for a moment. Isn't it excess carbohydrates that Dr. Robert Atkins, and Dr. Barry Sears (*Enter The Zone*) and other diet gurus, insist have caused the increase in obesity here in the U.S?

By taking control, reducing or eliminating many of the non-fatburning foods from your diet, you will be able to strike the match that ignites your body's natural fatburning mechanism. The key is to eat a variety of fatburning foods in moderation. Consistent small meals, severaltimes a day, will help keep your fatburning furnace burning on high. To do this, however, your fatburning furnace needs a constant source of fuel — food.

Note: *Please do not forget this simple principle. Moderation, frequency and a variety of your fatburning foods are crucial. Consuming any foods, especially fats and carbohydrates in excess of body need, will cause the body to store fat. It is also a myth that* *protein will not make you fat. Remember any food in excess will cause fat storage! Moderation is the key.*

Adding fatburning supplements

By applying the basic principles cited above, you will facilitate the resetting of your metabolic capacity. In this way, you are actually restoring the health and the fatburning potential of your body, through chemistry and the organizing power of nature. In the long run, this is exactly what you want — an internal fatburning thermostat that is on and kept in good working order.

Adding natural fatburning supplements to complement your new eating pattern can really shift your natural fatburning capacity into high gear. As with your food offerings, there are many choices. You are not locked into taking one supplement although you may select a product designed to focus on a special problem; for instance, Metabolife 356 for metabolism; or Satietrol, a fiber-based program designed as an appetite suppressant.

My personal choices of fatburning supplements, which are part of my everyday existence and lifestyle, are as follows.

- L-Carnitine
- A Multiple-Enzyme Formula
- Chromium
- Alpha-Lipore Acid
- Co-Q10
- A multiple fiber formula

I have a family history of blood sugar abnormalities that spans several generations and still plagues most of my living first line relatives. Many of the fatburning supplements listed help me to control my weight and also serve a very important second purpose. They help regulate blood sugar levels. To date, I am the only living person in my family who hasn't had any problems related to blood sugar. I use all these supplements in a combination formula, but you may find only one or two that work well for you. The bottom line here — you can win without diet drugs!

Many natural supplements are used synergistically (combining substances together). The active "chemicals" come packaged with beneficial counterparts (co-factors). These agents in many cases have the capability to ameliorate (to make better or more tolerable) any side effects that chemical combinations may have as separate entities. It is these phenomena and safety features that make natural fatburners the better choice. In a society that has become enormously dependent on drug therapy, many health advocates recommend re-thinking our position on the use of drug remedies to treat everyday common or non-life threatening ailments. Dr. Andrew Weil, M.D. one of the country's most well-known medical experts and leading proponent of alternative medicine says "we'll see a greater self-reliance in this new millennium. People will learn to manage and prevent disease on their own rather than seek immediate treatment."[14]

Of primary importance for choosing a weight-loss program (and especially when using diet drugs) as stated by Serena Gordon a DrKoop.com (former U.S. Surgeon General) health correspondent, "weight loss medication (and or supplements, for that matter) are only as good as the lifestyle changes that individuals are willing to make."[15]

Ten Fatburning Principles to Live By

The most powerful course of action to ensure you will succeed without diet drugs is to change your habits, not to focus on dieting. Devise a plan of action — a simple plan that will keep you focused on increasing your metabolism. For example:

1. Don't skip meals (eliminate starvation tactics);
2. Balance your intake of fats, carbohydrates and protein;
3. Eat only healthy snacks;
4. Drink plenty of water (8 to 10 glasses daily);
5. Consume smaller meals (eat 5 to 6 times a day);
6. Engage in some exercise or aerobic activity daily;
7. Get plenty of rest;
8. Do not skip breakfast;
9. Do not eat a full meal before bedtime;
10. Love thyself – be positive – take charge.

---

[1] Silver Sage Reduction Products brochure, Draper, UT, 1997.

[2] Eisenberg, D.M. et.al. "Unconventional Medicine in the United States," The New England Journal of Medicine, 1993, 328:246-52.

[3] Drake, D., Uhlman, M., *Making Medicine Making Money,* Andrew and McMeel Publishing, NY, 1993.

[4] "U.S. Weight Loss Market. Year 2001 Status Report," 3-01-01, Marketdata.com

[5] abcnews.go.com/sections/business/The Street/diet00626.html.

[6] King, J.S., "Retailers Gain Sales With Natural Weight Loss Aids," Whole Foods, Plainfield, NJ, March 1994, p.37-46.

[7] "U.S. Weight Loss Market. Year 2001 Status Report," 3-01-01, Marketdata.com

[8] Healthwatch, "Hot Diet Pills Are Prescription For Complications and Disappointment," Let's Live Mag., Los Angeles CA, April 1997, p.23.

[9] Rogers, S., "How the Sick Get Sicker Quicker Without Nutritional Supplements," Let's Live, #70 Vol. 62, Jan. 1994: 44-47.

[10] Diamond, Harvey, Diamond, Marilyn, *Fit For Life*, Warner Books, NY, 1985.

[11] Ibid.

[12] Kleiner, S.M., *Power Eating*, Human Kinetics, Champaign IL, 1998.

[13] Martlew, G., Electrolytes: *The Spark of Life,* Murdock, FL, Natures Publishing, LTD., 1994, p. 52.

[14] Weil A., *Health and Healing,* Houghton-Mifflin Company, Boston MA, 1995.

[15] Gordon, S., "A Magic Bullet For Weight Loss?" DrKoop.com, Aug. 8, 2001.

Chapter Six

Supplementation for Weight-Loss Programs

> *Numerous vitamins and pharmaceutical companies are now selling weight control products based on anti-fat nutrients. These products usually consist of multi-nutrients. While you can obtain a measure of success by using just one special nutrient or category of nutrients, your results can be enhanced by using a variety of anti-fat nutrients.*
>
> **Dr. Dallas Clouatre, Ph.D.,**
> *University of California, Berkley*
> *Anti-Fat Nutrients[1]*

Now that you have a basic knowledge concerning the biological rudiments of dieting and why dieting in the tradition sense is outmoded, please keep in mind that the goal of any good weight loss program should focus on long-term health versus a mere loss of a few pounds. Your weight and fat loss program as we learned in earlier chapters should focus on:

1. your fat-to-pound ratio;
2. curbing and controlling your appetite;
3. focusing on long-term health maintenance;
4. providing a constant flow of balanced nutrients;
5. maintaining existing energy levels;
6. being psychologically rewarding;
7. encouraging long-term habitual tendencies toward fat reduction and muscle building;
8. promoting the elimination of poor dietary habits;
9. changing sedentary lifestyles.

The purpose of this chapter is to give you an overview of some of the most popular natural products that can help sustain the health of your body, and assist in fighting fat as well. I would, however, like to emphasize that any fat-fighting properties of the supplements do not constitute magic weight loss pills, and should be used in conjunction with a sound exercise and nutritional program.

As you review this section of the book you will find many variations of fatburners that you will be able to use interchangeably that will help you achieve these goals safely, effectively and naturally. Some of the fatburners will help you lose pounds, while some will focus on inches. Some will assist you in slowing down absorption of fats while others will help you reduce cholesterol levels, prevent fatty deposits from clogging up your arteries, and some will help you burn fat stores more efficiently, that your body will use as fuel versus fat storage. You do not need a doctor's prescription to use these natural supplements. They are not drugs, they are classified as food supplements. The beauty in this approach is that you can augment your newfound eating patterns and experiment with various combinations of products tailored to your individual needs. Results can vary from person to person, due to individual response time.

There is no fear of moving one category of product into another or the cross-usage of two or three different categories. Always follow label instructions and be consistent with usage. As you reach your goals without sabotaging your health, you can go on and off these natural fatburners as your lifestyle and changing health dictates. You are in total control of your body. Have fun and use this life-long guide to educate yourself on the many natural fatburners you have at your disposal. If you are taking prescription medication, check with your doctor before you start, and remember:

*The direction in which education starts a man or woman will determine his or her future life, **and health!***

Plato

These natural supplements and protocols may actually enhance many of the body's inborn metabolic processes. "When the human physiology metabolizes a plant remedy, it actually metabolizes the organizing power of nature which the plant has transmitted into material form. In this simple way, the human physiology responds to and is governed by the physiology of nature, resulting in the harmonizing of the body and mind of human life with the body and mind of nature."[2]

The plant researchers who wrote the *Naturopathic Handbook of Herbal Formulas*, believe that the health and balance of the body is restored by chemistry and nature's organizing power. This is the way we were designed to work. You have at your disposal many safe alternatives and natural weight-loss aids that enhance body processes. Individual drugs are often re-marketed for use in treating symptoms other than their original design. Combining several of these drugs to increase their effectiveness (as was the case with Fen-phen) may not be safe and can have lethal consequences. *(See Appendix A for further information.)*

Consider the history of pharmacological anti-obesity drugs as cited by Dr. Caroline M. Apovian, M.D. who serves as Medical Director of the Program for Weight Management at Harvard Medical School in Boston, Massachusetts. Because of the increasing problem of obesity in the United States, Dr. Apovian argues that there is greater pharmacological incentive to produce new anti-obesity drugs and appetite suppressants. She correlates the similar historical track record of death and illness from obesity drugs with recent fen-phen disaster.[3] Current estimates by the World Health Organization puts the use of plant-based medicines by the world's population at 75 to 80 percent. This due in part to lower cost, minimal side-effects, a safer track record, and comparable results to their drug counterparts.

The following is a compilation of safer and more effective methods to sustain health while losing unwanted pounds. To my knowledge, these products do not have the possible dangerous consequences, as did Fen-Phen, current diet drugs and surgical procedures. You will find this section divided into seven different categories. Please choose the category or product you feel meets your immediate needs.

A note of caution: *While natural weight loss components are relatively safe and have a long history of use, please check with your healthcare professional before mixing any herbal or other preparations with any prescribed medication you may be taking. Pregnant and lactating women also should consult their healthcare professional before starting or using any supplement plan or protocol.*

Adjunct Compounds

Acidophilus
This natural bacteria is vital to good colon health and should be a primary supplement on your list. Maintaining a healthy colon is also essential to good liver function. Acidophilus can prevent the colon from unloading excess toxins into the liver from the mesenteric vein, which forces waste materials from the colon to the portal vein and into the liver. This will also aid the liver in its job of

handling fats for proper metabolism and utilization. Certain strains of bacteria in the colon have been implicated with intestinal toxemia. Bacteria such as that of the clostridium family can metabolize unabsorbed nutrients or food by-products like bile or fatty acids and cholesterol, and transmute them into deadly carcinogens. In addition to protecting us from harmful bacteria, acidophilus is involved with the proper transmutation of nutrients into their health-building components. These nutrients include the all-important B vitamins, which assist in metabolism. Researchers now know that all species have their own internal biological keys and micro-ecosystems. Because of this, acidophilus must be of human origin to maximize its utilization in the human colon.

Citrus Aurantium

This is a natural digestive aid derived from the bitter "Seville" orange fruit. It has been used nutritionally for thousands of years. Researchers have learned the Citrus Aurantium induces thermogenesis (the act of speeding up the rate at which the body uses calories), without adversely affecting blood pressure and heart rate. It can be used as an alternative to Ephedra, to increase the body's ability to metabolize stored body fat and provide a greater amount of energy.[4]

CLA

In scientific circles, CLA is short for Conjugated Linoleic Acid. This free fatty acid (a good fat) is not saturated and is vital to the body's ability to retain muscle tone and reduce body fat. Naturally found in dairy products, meat, sunflower oil and safflower oil, this fatty acid is causing quite a stir, because of its fatburning capabilities. However, to get adequate daily quantities of this important compound you would have to consume three pounds of hamburger, twenty-five slices of American cheese, or a half-gallon of ice cream. In a study at the University of Wisconsin, test subjects were given CLA at levels of 0.6 percent of their dietary intake. Results indicated that body fat percentages declined by 46 percent, while lean muscle increase by 9 percent. Suggested dosage as recommended by these researchers is 1 to 2 grams of CLA daily.[5]

While researchers have yet to find out exactly how this natural agent assist the body, they do know that it modulates the metabolism of fat, discourages fat storage with the help of an enzyme called lipoprotein lipase and scavenges fat cells.[6]

CoQ10

Because of mounting evidence, researchers contend that a vitamin-like substance, similar in structure to Vitamin K and Vitamin E, may have a positive influence in reducing a wide range of ailments. Acting as a co-enzyme, Q10 (called CoQ10 for short), is found everywhere in the body. Because of its unique existence, scientists began referring to the entire class of CoQ's as "ubiquinones," coined from the Latin word *ubique*, meaning everywhere.

CoQ$_{10}$ is technically 2.3-dimethoxy-5-methyl-6-decarprenyl-1, 4-benzoquinone, or 2.3-dimethoxy-5-methyl-6-[3-methyl-2-butenylenkakis-(3-methyl-2-butenylene)]1;4-benzoquininone. Microorganisms have CoQ as 6,7, or 9 isoprenoid units (CoQ6, CoQ7, CoQ9). Mammalian (any group of vertebrate animals, including human beings, that feeds its young with milk from the female mammary glands) CoQ is of the 10-unit isoprenoid type, which gives way to its distinction and its application. The isoprenoid units may have similar functions but, because of the nature of their germane, they can show differences in some properties, such as the different control mechanisms in a given cell. The structure of all CoQ molecules resembles a head with a tail. The tail can have up to 12 repeating units. The body manufactures only one type of CoQ, with a tail of 10 repeated units, for which it is named.

In 1957, CoQ10 was first extracted from animal tissue. Researchers found that CoQ10 had the ability to remove oxygen from a biologically active molecule. The importance of this reaction is critical, due to the fact that a lack of oxygen can produce a decline in cellular energy, while too much can cause the formation of toxic elements allowing conditions conducive for diseased states to exist and flourish.

The discovery of this unique substance came from Japan. Further, clinical trials conducted by Dr. Karl Folkers, of the University of Texas confirmed the efficacy of its ability to slow down many degenerative diseases. Dr. Folkers, known as the father of CoQ10 in the United States, also led the research team that discovered Vitamin B^{12} in 1948 and was one of the first researchers to synthesize Vitamin B^{6}. Dr. Folkers received the Priestley Medal, from the American Chemical Society in 1986, its highest award, for his research on Co-enzyme, Q10.

Based on clinical trials conducted by Dr. Folkers and other researchers, CoQ10 has been established to be essential in:

• having favorable effects on muscular metabolism in patients with chronic lung disease and insufficient blood-oxygen stores;

• the bio-energy generation process known as the Kreb's cycle, the common pathway in the conversion of the energy produced from the food we eat;

• improving respiratory energy production in heart cells;

• normalizing blood pressure;

• neutralizing the damaging effects of free radical destruction, implicated in over 60 age-related degenerative diseases;

• acting as a catalyst in the chain of chemical reactions that create energy needed by cells to stay alive;

Note: This process is critical in reference to how efficiently the body's natural metabolic fatburning processes ignite. Researchers in Belgium found that in 50 percent of individuals classified as obese, the mechanism or catalytic action of CoQ10 production was insufficient. The problem is that under normal circumstances the body naturally steps up its energy output when a meal is consumed. In many overweight individuals this response is severely compromised.

• protecting the heart from damage due to a heart attack, as well as reduce the amount of tissue damage that occurs during open-heart surgery;

• reducing periodontal disease, diabetes, deafness and impaired immunity;

• diminishing the toxic effects of beta-blockers, chemotherapeutic agents, and psychotrophic drugs; and

• accelerating the thermogenetic process, thus assisting the body in its ability to burn stored body fat.

Like Vitamin E, CoQ10 can help protect against "fat peroxidation." Peroxidized fats are essentially rancid fats. In this form, these fats suppress the immune system, become mutagens, carcinogens, cross-linkers, and compounds like hydrogen peroxide. These compounds will accelerate aging.[7] Furthermore, in a study by Van Gaal, 100 milligrams of CoQ10 was given to a control group on a restricted diet. After nine weeks, the non-control group had low levels of the enzyme without having been administered CoQ10, but were also on a restrictive diet. There was a reduction of 13.5 pounds (controlled) versus 5.8 (non-controlled). The researchers of this study concluded that a combination of a low-calorie diet and supplementation of CoQ10 may result in weight loss superior to that obtained from restricted diet alone.[8]

No serious side effects have been reported with long-term clinical use of CoQ10. With all the overwhelming evidence to the effectiveness of this substance, supplementation of this compound can prove to be very beneficial since it has been shown that foods lose CoQ10 content with processing and storage. CoQ10 benefits a number of individuals such as heart patients, diabetics and the clinically obese.

Pyruvate

After twenty-five years of research into the efficiency of this substance, pyruvate is now available as a supplement. Data has confirmed that pyruvate is effective as both a weight- and fat-loss product. Dr. Ronald T. Stanko, M.D., of the Gastroenterologic and Clinical Nutrition Division at the University of Pittsburgh Medical Center, found that obese women who were given pyruvate for three weeks lost 37 percent more weight (13 versus 9.5 lbs.) and 48 percent more fat (8.8 versus 5.9 lbs.). Dr. Stanko concluded from this study that the 48 percent increase in fat loss could be seen or converted into a loss of nearly an extra pound of body fat per week.[9]

As discussed previously, the problem associated with on-and-off dieting is increased fat storage. Some of the most promising data on pyruvate suggests that it can drastically decrease or impair both weight and fat that accumulate due to excessive caloric intake. In other words, pyruvate may provide a natural means to help those individuals prone to on-and-off binge eating, thus helping to keep weight off permanently.

Furthermore, recent data has confirmed the fact that after several continuous days of a low-calorie diet, liver ATP (Adenosine-Tri-Phosphate, the body's main fuel source) drops to sub-par levels. This occurrence causes a reduction in body temperature and inhibits fat loss. Although there are many compounds that are able to sustain liver ATP, pyruvate is believed to be far superior in this respect.

Creatine

This compound is part of our body's natural energy cycle and is made from the amino acids arginine, methionine and glycine. Its chemical name is Methylguanido-acetic Acid. Manufactured in the liver, as well as the pancreas and kidneys, it is transported by the blood, and utilized mainly in muscle cells. Creatine is derived largely from creatine phosphate in muscle. Creatine is intimately involved with ATP (Adenosine-tri-phosphate) — our main energy molecule. It is naturally supplied to our body for energy to assist in muscular contraction. Creatine is mainly derived from consuming red meat. Changes in blood levels of creatine concentration can occur due to changes in muscle mass. Anecedotal reference as well as scientific studies have reported that creatine:

- helps build lean body mass;
- increases energy levels, thus increasing work-load; and
- speeds recovery (muscle soreness).

Researchers contend that creatine promotes muscle growth because of its ability to enhance the body's use of protein (our main building blocks). In addition to the above, when more creatine is shuttled into the muscle cell, more water is also brought in with it. This concept — natural shuttle service and consequent utilization of nutrients by the muscle cell — is known as cell volumizing. For instance, when muscle cells become overly saturated with water and other nutrients, scientists believe the body signals the muscle to use protein more efficiently to build muscle, and increases glycogen (stored fuel) for energy utilization.

Due to the nature and the amount of creatine, serum (blood) concentration levels vary. The normal range for serum creatine in the adult is about 60-120 umol/1. According to Dr. William Marshall, the day-to-day variation in an individual can actually be much lower than this range.[10] The natural manufacture of creatine by the body is usually not enough to meet demands, and therefore slows down muscle protein breakdown or catabolism (when body breaks down its own muscle tissue to meet building and energy needs). Researchers have found that ingesting five grams of creatine four times a day for a period of four to five days and thereafter, maintaining a dosage of five grams once a day, led to an average increase of about 25 percent of creatine in the muscle. The practice of advance loading to increase and maintain creatine concentrations was pioneered by Hultman and Colleagues at the Department of Clinical Chemistry at the Karolinska Institute in Sweden.[11] There are presently available forms of creatine serum (liquid) that do not require a loading phase dose.

Lecithin

Lecithin is a naturally occurring substance that acts as an emulsifier. An emulsifer could be compared to your heavy-duty washing powder, which is capable of breaking down dirt, grit and grime. Lecithin works the same way in the body except that its actions are towards fat. Lecithin actually helps to dissolve fat and cholesterol, as well as preventing accumulation of excess fat in the liver. The richest natural sources of lecithin are the B-vitamins choline and inositol.

While lecithin is found in every living cell in the body, its highest concentration is in the vital organs, such as the brain, heart, the liver and the kidneys. Since the liver is the primary site where lipids (fat) are metabolized, lecithin is of vital importance to keeping your body's natural fatburning cycle on high. Research conducted at major educational institutions such as New York University, Northwestern University and the University of Chicago, indicates that lecithin promotes the breakdown of deposits of fatty materials and cholesterol deposits in certain organs.[12]

Note: *While there is no (as of yet) established RDA for lecithin, daily dosages most often used range from 500 to 1,000 mg.*[13]

Water

While water itself is not a supplement, I do consider it an accessory compound, crucial to helping you achieve your weight- and fat-loss goals. Water is the essence of life and most of your internal makeup (60 percent) is of water. Water is the medium your body uses to help flush your kidneys to assist with the elimination of waste byproducts. For fatburning purposes, according to Dr. Ellington Darden, Ph.D., former Director of Research for Nautilus Sports Medical Industries, the body will expend 123 calories of body heat a day to raise the temperature of ice-cold water at 40°F to 98.6° F.[14] According to Dr. Darden, by consuming about 128 ounces of ice cold water a day you can drop a pound a month, and that doesn't even take into consideration all the calories you will burn sprinting to the bathroom.

Amino Acids

Throughout the ages, scientists have sought to find a way to reduce the wear and tear of the human structure. We are essentially protein beings. Our skin, hair, nails, teeth, bones, arteries and veins are all made from protein. Protein is known as the building blocks of life.

Although vital to our very existence, the protein from the steak you ate last night or the garden salad you had at lunch today must be broken down into smaller pieces — the amino acids which are the end product of protein digestion. So vital are these substances that the body seeks to maintain what is called a "free amino acid pool." According to Dr. Francis Nettl, M.D., former Director of Exercise and Rehabilitation Medicine, US Navy, San Diego, CA, the amino acid pool can be understood if you imagine it as a small tank or reservoir. Within this reservoir, the amino acids that are present help your metabolism repair and build lean muscle tissue.[15] In the absence of proper metabolic processes, the body will break down or catabolize skeletal muscle tissue to provide amino acids.

Present knowledge has isolated 22 amino acids. Of these, eight are considered to be *essential*, meaning the body cannot manufacture them and therefore they must be supplied via the diet. The other fourteen, referred to as *non-essential*, can be manufactured by the body. This distinction is labeled as a misnomer by health officials, because biologically, all 22 are essential for optimal health. The synopsis that follows gives a general overview of the many popular amino acids in reference to the metabolism and breakdown of body fats, thus encouraging lean muscle growth.

Note: *Eating six to eight times a day will avoid the auto-catabolism as described above. The steady stream of food factors will help stabilize blood sugar as well as supply the body with substances that can be biotransmuted to amino acids, helping to maintain proper amino acid pool ratio's. Obesity researchers have concluded that this is the best method to keep your internal fires burning and metabolizing fat properly.*[16]

- *L-Carnitine:* In order for body fat to be utilized as fuel, it must first be freed from the fat cells where it is stored. This process is known as lypolysis. Physiologists contend that there is a direct correlation to the type and extent of vigorous programs that stimulate lypolysis. Researchers have corroborated the fact that L-carnitine, a non-essential amino acid is a key substance that liberates the mobilization of fats. Although we manufacture L-carnitine, some amounts are however very appreciable.

   There is evidence that improper carnitine levels inside the cell cause fatty acids to be metabolized very slowly. This can cause an excessive buildup within the cell and on the areas surrounding it, which can lead to elevated blood fat and triglycerides (the most common fat in food). Data suggests that 1000 to 3000 mg of carnitine daily are needed to improve fat metabolism and to reduce blood triglycerides.[17] When sufficient L-carnitine is present, the body's ability to break down fats into fatty acids is enhanced. Using the analogy of a shuttle bus, these fatty acids are transported into the mitochondria, (the power plants of the cell) where they are burned as fuel and used to produce energy.

L-Carnitine and Ketosis: Dr. Jeffrey Bland describes ketosis as a state in which low carbohydrate levels exist.[18] When this occurs, proponents of this state (known as the ketogenic diet), insist that if our body does not contain appreciable amounts of carbohydrates to draw on for energy, the body must resort to an alternate source for fuel, namely stored body fat. If this diet is not monitored, especially in diabetic patients, this ketone body may cause the blood to become "acidic," possibly generating excessive urinary loss of vital electrolytes as the body seeks to eliminate the unused calories. If left unchecked, this condition may become life threatening. Researchers now know that L-Carnitine via its ability to foster proper metabolism of fats, actually prevents the accumulation of ketone bodies.

- *Gaba:* Scientifically, gaba is known as gamma amino butyric acid. Gaba is widely used for its ability to combat stress, reduce anxiety and for its natural tranquilizing affect. Mounting evidence however, shows that gaba plays a major role in the release of GH (Growth Hormone), which greatly shifts the body's fat-burning ability from "Park" to "Turbo-drive"! As we have learned, growth hormone has a profound effect on our body's ability to maintain muscle and reduce body fat.

- *Phenylalanine:* Phenylalanine helps suppress appetite by its natural action of being converted in the body into neurotransmitters. Neurotransmitters help carry signals from the brain cells to other parts of the body. According to Dr. William H. Lee, a renowned amino acid researcher, when there is a lot of L-phenylalanine present, signals between brain cells become stronger.[19]

The two brain chemicals L-phenylalanine produces are norepinephrine and dopamine. Classified as excitatory transmitters these are the brain chemicals which make us feel good about ourselves. Furthermore, norepinephrine stimulates the release of the hormone cholecystokinin (CCK). When CCK is produced and released, it signals the brain that the stomach is full and needs no more food, thus making you feel full. Recommended dose is 100 to 500 mg in the morning on an empty stomach, to offset competition for absorption especially that of protein.[20] This amino acid can be found in an L-form or DL-form. You want the L-form. Please note that DL-phenylaline and L-phenylaline is different from phenylalanine (aspartame), which has been reported to have negative effects on the brain and cause headaches in some people.

   Note: *Persons who use MAO inhibitors (which include certain antidepressants), have high blood pressure, the genetic disease "PKU" (Phenylketonia) should not use phenylalanine. PKU is a benign condition that is caused by a metabolic block, which can cause severe mental retardation.*[21]

- *L-Orinithine, L-Argine and L-Lysine:* These three amino acids are touted for their ability to release growth hormone, which is stimulated by the pituitary gland and called the master gland (because it regulates the actions of other glands). It can alter your body's muscle to fat ratio (which alters fat). Growth hormone promotes maintenance and building of muscle as well as burning fat for your body's energy needs. Combinations of these three amino acids are one of the most widely used ingredients in commercial products to stimulate growth hormone release.[22]

   Growth Hormone releasers are best utilized by the body when taken on an empty stomach, preferably one hour before bedtime (as the body's natural release of GH takes place 90 minutes after falling asleep). Growth hormone release also occurs during intense exercise therefore it may be useful to take these amino acids prior to workouts. Co-factors that enhance GH release are vitamin B^6, panthotenic acid (Vitamin B^5) and choline.

   Note: *Since these amino acids are directly linked to the actions of the pitutary gland and its release of growth hormone, it is not recommended for children (unless specified by a physician) or lactating women.*

- *Branch Chain Amino Acids (BCAA's):* Leucine, isoleucine and valine are called branch-chained aminos due to the fact that they look like branch-like side chains of atoms, much like the branches on a tree. Approximately thirty-five percent of BCAA's are found in muscle tissue. These amino acids play a critical role in the preservation of lean muscle tissue, especially during high-intensity weight training. The body uses the branch-chained aminos as an indirect energy supply for the muscles by converting them to glucose in the liver (the process of gluconeogenesis). Research also has confirmed Leucine's ability to stimulate the release of growth hormone. Scientists contend that there is no group of amino acids more important in accelerating muscle growth as well cultivating its maintenance.[23]

To assess the benefits of BCAA supplementation, Mowier and his co-workers studied a group of wrestlers placed on a hypocaloric, hypocaloric high-protein, hypocaloric BCAA and hypocaloric low-protein diet. Although every category of dieters as specified had significant loss of total bodyweight, the greatest loss of 8.8 pounds occurred in the hypocaloric BCAA group.

Additionally, all groups had a loss of body fat composition, but the BCAA's groups loss of 3.7 percent fat was higher than the others, suggesting that supplementation with BCAA's had increased benefits.[24]

Note: *Branch-chain amino acids are a special breed in that they are synthesized directly in the muscle, in contrast to most amino acids, which are metabolized in the gut.*

5-HTP

The major action of the drug Fen-Phen was to increase levels of serotonin (5HT) in the brain. There however, is one major draw back. According to Dr. Judith J. Wurtman of MIT, the fact remains that while Fen-Phen/Redux-enhanced serotonin activity in the brain, they had no effect on the brain's supply of serotonin.[25] Serotonin, an important neurotransmitter which is linked to a number of brain functions is crucial to impulses between nerve cells that relate to weight control, insomnia, obsessive-compulsive disorders as well as eating disorders that lead to obesity.[26]

Serotonin is produced from trypotophan in the body. L-trytophan is the raw material the brain uses to make serotonin, melatonin and niacin (vitamin B^3). Scientist's have now confirmed that you can increase levels of serotonin in the brain by supplementation of its metabolic precursor, 5-hydroxytryptophan (5-HTP).[27] When taken up by the cell, tryptophan is converted to 5-HTP, which is then biologically transmuted or converted into 5HT (serotonin). It is this conversion, which is important in the function of selective serotonin re-uptake inhibitors such as Prozac, Paxil and Zoloft, often prescribed to persons wanting to lose weight. Unfortunately, like Fen-Phen and Redux, these drugs do not produce any serotonin (5HT). Serotonin is produced from trytophan within the body.[28]

A placebo-controlled study by J. Blundell in 1991 at the University of Leeds, Italy, involved 20 obese patients, who were administered 100 milligrams a day of 5HTP. The results revealed that they lost considerable amounts of weight, had reduced carbohydrate intake and better appetite control than the placebo group. Current data validates 5-HTP's conversion of trytophan to serotonin.

When tryptophan-free amino acid mixtures were administered to patients on selective serotonin re-uptake inhibitors (SSRI) therapy, their clinical state worsened. This is due to the fact that with insufficient amounts of trypotophan to act upon by the brain, a decreased serotonin synthesis (less serotonin for SSRI's to interact with), suggests increasing dietary use of 5-HTP in the treatment of obesity. Researchers conclude that with the ability of 5-HTP (5-hydroxtryptophan) to increase serotonin, the variation of it is not likely to occur with 5-HTP supplementation.[29]

Note: *Tryptophan is found in relatively large quantities of bananas and milk. Since 1988 tryptophan supplements have been banned in the United States when the Food and Drug Administration (FDA) banned all tryptophan products due to a contaminated supply batch from manufactures in Japan. The FDA's provision does not apply to 5-HTP.*

Enzymes

Enzymes are a class of proteins serving as catalysts. Chemically, enzymes are agents that change the rate of a reaction without being consumed or changed by the reaction. In the absence of enzymes, many metabolic reactions would take an enormous amount of time to occur and the metabolic pathways would become congested much like rush hour traffic or a clogged sink. Enzyme-deficient individuals, who suffer from digestive problems, could see their condition escalate to liver and gallbladder dysfunction, heart and circulatory problems and weight gain. Digestive enzymes help to break down fats, carbohydrates and proteins into smaller units, thus preparing them for utilization by the body.

There are three classes of enzymes. *Metabolic* enzymes run our body, *digestive* enzymes digest our food, and *raw food enzymes* initiate food digestion. Digestive enzymes have only three main duties — to digest protein, carbohydrates and fats. Protease is an enzyme that digests protein, amylase digests carbohydrate, and lipase digests fat. There are different enzymes for different metabolic actions, and to break down food into smaller component parts (sugars to carbohydrates, fats to fatty acids, proteins to amino acids). This action (breakdown) takes place within the digestive system.[30]

Dr. Edward Howell, a pioneer in the medical applications of enzyme therapy states in his book, *Enzyme Nutrition: The Food Enzyme Concept*, that the easiest way to separate fat from its lipase enzyme is to destroy the lipase by cooking. Since enzymes are destroyed when exposed to extreme heat the fat, dislodged from its lipase companion, is forced to remain undigested for a period of two, three or more hours after it is swallowed thus contributing to our worries about cholesterol. To make matters worse, when commercial fat is consumed without its lipase companion, it interacts with the enzyme hydrochloric acid in the human stomach and may be left with a structural defect. Without sufficient quantities of lipase, the fat will not be properly digested in the intestine. This process, according to Dr, Howell, may have a direct bearing on the country's existing obesity problem.

Although many Americans have reduced their fat (especially saturated) intake, they are still getting fatter. Those of us who eat a majority of cooked foods have destroyed the enzymes that breakdown fats, carbohydrates and proteins. The body must now pick up the slack and produce the necessary enzymes for digestion. Although medical authorities some years ago considered this to be a continuous occurrence, researchers now know there is a marked decline in enzyme production as we age.

The problem of enzyme production and proper metabolism of fats is exacerbated by the Standard American Diet (SAD) which contains excessive fat and sugar consumption. This forces the body to borrow from a non-existent supply of trace minerals and enzymes every time we eat. Trace minerals in their electrolyte form (dissolved and broken down by the body), assist in the removal of undigested fats and other debris, and also help reduce cravings for refined sugars and carbohydrates, major culprits in your battle against the bulge. Additionally, trace minerals are intimately involved with proper protein metabolism and how the body uses protein to build new muscle tissue. Few of us have an ample reserve of trace minerals and enzymes to draw on, thereby leaving fats undigested. This fact is linked to increased obesity in this country and an increase of other maladies as well.

The risk to health lies in the fact that as we age, our body's production of enzymes begins to decline. Research scientists today contend that this diminishing production of enzymes opens the door for many disease states to exist and flourish. Dr. Joseph Weissman, M.D., an immunologist and assistant clinical professor at the University of California Medical School, states that staying healthy may correlate with the amount of enzymes in our bodies.[31] This is evidenced in the fact that cystic fibrosis, the most common lethal genetic disease in the United States strikes 1 out of every 2,500 Caucasians[32] and is caused by a deficiency of the enzymes, trypsin and lipase. Due to ongoing worldwide research, scientists now know that supplementing with enzymes has enormous therapeutic value for sustaining health and bodily metabolic processes.

As stated, lipase is the enzyme that helps the body break down fats, and assists in lipolysis (the chemical breakdown of body fat by enzymes, which results in stored body fat being used as fuel by the body.) Without adequate amounts of lipase in the body, fat will stagnate and cause weight gain. Dr. David Galton, at the School of Medicine, Tufts University, confirmed the above when he tested subjects weighing on average 230 pounds. From his research, he discovered that each and every participant was lacking in enzymes in their fatty tissue.[33]

The liver is one of our most essential organs because it manufacturers bile, essential for the digestion of fat. When the liver is unable to secrete enough bile, the fat is not completely digested. Not only is this detrimental to overall health, this isn't good for those on a weight- and fat-loss program. Also, fat not fully digested tend to leave a film of fat on other foods, thus making them difficult to digest.

Based on past and present research, health officials suggest the use of supplemental enzymes to aid in weight control, for digestive disorders and for general maintenance of health. This suggestion is strongly recommended for individuals over the age of 40. Dr. Howell also insists that if we take in more exogenous [outside] digestive enzymes, the body's full enzyme potential can be reached. This is due to the fact that more metabolic enzymes would be distributed for vital energy processes, as nature intended.[34]

Furthermore, while there still remains much controversy in relationship to oral enzyme therapy, Dr. Hans Kugler, author of

Slowing Down the Aging Process, states that current technology has proven enzymes can be absorbed orally.[35] This fact was corroborated by Dr. David Graham, Department of Medicine at Baylor College of Medicine, who discovered that commercially available oral pancreatic enzyme extracts were able to improve digestion and assimilation of protein and fat in people with pancreatic insufficiency.[36] The role of enzymes in a well-balanced exercise, weight and fat loss program has enormous potential in the treatment of the clinically obese patient. Conversely, there exist many different biochemical pathways. Enzymes are believed to be the biological keys that keep bodily processes functioning at peak levels. Once the body has exhausted its supply of enzymes, systems shut down, resulting in depressed metabolic processes up to and including the fatburning process. As such, current data suggests that continued daily application of multiple enzymes would be of benefit to a sound weight management program.

Food Factors

In 1965, an early pioneer of nutritional medicine made the following statement, which is paraphrased here: Today we are not only in the "Atomic Age," but also the "Antibiotic Age." Unhappily, I also consider this the "Dark Age of Medicine," an age in which many of my colleagues, when confronted with a patient, then decide which pink or purple or blue pill to prescribe for the patient. This is not in my opinion, the practice of medicine. Far too many of these new "miracle" drugs are introduced with fanfare and then revealed as lethal in character, to be silently discarded for newer and more powerful drugs. These sentiments are echoed by Dr. Henry G. Bieler, M.D., who advises the use of proper food instead of drugs to prevent and cure disease and covers many key areas related to obesity in *Food Is Your Best Medicine*, which serves as a cornerstone to the following text. Current research has proved without a doubt that there is a direct relationship to what you eat, how it is absorbed, and resultant health.[37]

Utilizing foodstuffs to increase metabolic cycles has become common practice today. The discussion that follows covers some of those food factors used today to correct and treat the clinically obese, as well as maintain desired weight levels.

Essential Fatty Acids

Although we have repeatedly been told to avoid fat, health officials are beating a different drum. In our quest to reduce fat from our diets at all cost, data suggest that we have gone overboard. In fact, health experts are suggesting that this has contributed to our problem of obesity rather than diminish it, because of over-consumption of carbohydrates.[38]

For the last several years, many diet enthusiasts have recommended ultra-low-fat consumption (10%). The rational is that dietary fat, like single sugars, is easily converted into body fat. Proponents argue that the body uses up less energy (3 percent) storing fat calories as fat, than it does storing calories from carbohydrates (25 percent). Evidence continues to mount that shows the limiting of our intake of essential fatty acids actually encourages storage of body fat. The designation of essential refers to the fact that our bodies are incapable of making these fats. They must be supplied via dietary means. Saturated fats clog our arteries, and essential fatty acids need usually increases in relationship to increased saturated fat intake and carbohydrate consumption.

While reducing fat from the diet is a good idea for most Americans, Dr. Kevin Maki, Ph.D., of the Chicago Center for Clinical Research, maintains that we shouldn't exclude any food from our diet, including fat. Dr. Maki and colleagues found that when saturated fat intake was low, consuming red or white meat didn't raise cholesterol levels. This study suggests that fats offer some real benefits in weight- and fat-loss management. The problem seems to lie with the type of fat ingested and how much of which fat slows down the process of lipolysis which as stated previously, can be defined as splitting fat into component parts, namely fatty acids.[39]

The two essential fatty acids that must absolutely come from dietary sources are linoleic and linolenic acids. The National Research Council of the U.S. recommends that one percent of your fat intake come from essential fatty acids. Our advice is to consider reducing your saturated fat intake and increase your intake of essential fatty acids to five percent. The following are examples of essential fatty acids (the good fat):

- black currant oil
- borage oil
- evening primrose oil
- flax oil or seed (ground)
- olive oil
- omega 3s (fish oils)
- safflower oil
- soybean oil
- sunflower oil
- wheat germ oil

Medium Chain Tryglicerides (MCT)

This highly charged fat is used extensively because it enters the bloodstream and is immediately converted to glucose, releasing energy to the body. Besides supplying you with quick energy for your exercise or workout routine, MCTs come with an added benefit. Obesity researchers suggest exchanging MCT oil for starchy carbohydrates. This change will increase your body's thermogenic capabilities, twofold. According to Maggie Greenwood Robinson, nutritionist and author,[40] when you cut back on your carbohydrate consumption, you decrease the release of insulin thus allowing the hormone glucagon to step up its action. Glucagon is the hormone that acts like a key to unlock fat cells and encourage their use as fuel. Insulin has an opposite effect — it locks up fat cells and encourages fat storage. MCT oil used in this capacity will help speed up metabolism and your ability to burn body fat as well as preserve lean muscle tissue.

Fiber

Although health officials have called for more fiber to become a daily part of the American diet, people do not consume the recommended twenty-five grams a day. About three to five tablespoons of bran would be optimal for good intestinal function. We also advise following the USDA (United States Department of Agriculture) guidelines of consuming 2-4 four servings of fruit and 3 to 5 servings of vegetables daily. Current data puts the average daily American dietary intake of fiber at eleven grams.

Dietary fiber adds bulk to the system and assists with very important digestive and eliminative functions. Fiber, which is basically the structural material that makes up plants, is not absorbed into the bloodstream. For example, soluble fiber (those capable of being dissolved or liquefied) such as barley, oats, legumes and pectin (apples, fruits), bind with cholesterol and other digestive byproducts thus inhibiting their assimilation. The insoluble fiber (those incapable of being dissolved) such as cellulose, hemicellulose (bran, vegetables, grains) and lignin (whole grains) help create moisture and bulk. This reduces transit time, fatty deposits and other byproducts in the alimentary canal. As cited in an earlier study at the USDA's Human Research Center in Beltsville, Maryland, researchers concluded that fiber interferes with the absorption of fat into the intestines. These researchers state that persons who eat a high-fat, low-fiber diet will absorb 98 out of every 100 grams of fat consumed.

As an aid to weight loss, fiber can slow down the absorption of fat, and help curb your appetite when consumed about thirty minutes prior to eating. Dr. Rosemary Newman, Ph.D., R.N., a registered dietician and professor of Foods and Nutrition at Montana State University in Bozeman, insists that high-fiber foods are very low in calories and fat. For these reasons, they should be a major part of any weight loss plan. Researchers now know that a diet providing 25 to 35 grams a day of soluable and insoluable fibers can lower blood glucose levels in healthy individuals. Current data suggests that daily intake of optimal amounts of fiber can reduce blood cholesterol by as much as 19 to 26 percent.[41]

One type of newly discovered fiber is Chitosan. Chitosan is made from chitin, an amino polysaccharide fiber found in the shells of crawfish, lobster and other shellfish. Data indicates that large dosages of chitosan may reduce fat absorption. This occurs through a process called "deacetylation" which refers to the removal of acetyl groups. Marketers of this marine fiber product claim that the above process improves solubility of the fiber. In their experiments with Chitosan, Kaneuchi and co-workers reported that it reduces fat absorption by dissolving in the stomach, and biotransmutting into a gel structure. This enables Chitosan to trap and engulf fat in the intestines, in essence blocking its absorption.[42]

In addition, when dietary fiber is agitated (fermented) by the flora within the intestines, short chain fatty acids are formed. David Kritchevsky, a researcher at the world-renowned Wistar Institute of Anatomy and Biology in Philadelphia, PA, maintains that valuable actions are exhibited in this process with acetic, proprionic and butyric acids, all short chain fatty acids (SCFA). Propriorate and acetate are transported to the liver and broken down to produce energy. Butyrate provides energy for the cells within the colon, thus promoting growth of healthy bacteria.[43]

Due to the dynamic action of fiber within the digestive tract, many naturopaths and nutritionists recommend in today's environment of highly processed foods that intake of daily dietary fiber be increased to 50 grams. The word fiber first appeared on the English language scene in 1907, and has evolved into a nutrition concept in its own right. But only in the last decade has it gained acceptance among medical authorities.

Note: *There is evidence that excessive amounts of fiber may interfere with the uptake of certain minerals. Data suggest that fiber in foods will not cause the above mishap. However, large amounts of additional fiber may cause mineral imbalances.[44] Because of this, it is not recommended that you take your vitamin and mineral supplements at the same time you take your fiber supplements.*

Glucomannan

This fiber, which is extracted from the tubers of the Amorphophallus Konjac root, is known for its ability to reduce serum (blood) lipids (fats) and stabilize blood sugar. By forming a gel in the intestinal tract, glucomannan gives you a feeling of fullness. Because of this action, it is advisable to drink plenty of water when using this product.

Olive Oil

Although oils are considered as fats, some are better than others and are easier on the digestive system. One such oil is olive oil. A staple in Italy and the cornerstone of the "Mediterranean Diet," olive oil has a history as a beneficial food with relatively low risk of cardiovascular disease. This is due in part to the fact that dietary olive oil stimulates the pancreas to secrete bicarbonate and digestive enzymes, and the gallbladder to release bile. When the intake of dietary olive oil is increased, total content of bile acids in the intestines increase. In turn, this stimulation of bile initiates the release of enzymes from the pancreas, which assists in the breakdown of fat.

Lemons

In naturopathic circles the addition of lemons (or limes) in conjunction with a daily tablespoon of olive oil is ideal for stimulating proper breakdown of fats and to reverse cholestasis (the stoppage of bile flow). They also help to cleanse and neutralize fatty deposits due to sluggish liver and gallbladder function.

Naturopathic practitioners suggest mixing ten lemons in two quarts of water (sweeten with natural honey or stevia) and along with ¼ teaspoon of olive oil, drink one glass every two hours for three days.[45] Known as the "Master Cleanser" or "The Lemonade Diet," this program has been shown to be very effective up to ten days or more. For severe cases of congested, clogged or toxic liver, forty-day intervals may be needed.[46] When obesity has become a problem and better assimilation and digestion is needed, the "lemon diet" three to four times a year will help keep fatburning cycles on high.[47]

Soy

In the last decade, there has been an explosion of information concerning the benefits of soy. No less than 38 controlled clinical studies appearing in the New England Journal of Medicine have examined the link between soy and its reductional ability on cholesterol and triglycerides.[48]

In Asia, soybeans are used in over 400 different ways, according to Charles B. Heiser, Jr., in *Seed to Civilization,* as cited by Ruth Adams and Frank Murry in their exposé titled "Health Foods."[49] They are mentioned in Chinese literature as early as 1,000 years before Christ. The soybean is one of the richest, most nutritious foods in the world, being 11 percent protein and six percent oils.[50]

Soybeans contain a very high quality protein with an amino acid content almost equaling that of eggs and meat. In fact, soybeans are the only natural food that contains all the essential amino acids that the body needs to synthesize all the other amino acids. Additionally, Patricia Hausman, author of *Foods That Fight Cancer,* reminds us that soybeans have a moderate fat count. She contends that soybeans and other foods, such as lentils and navy beans, have protein contents that rival that of meat, poultry and fish. She suggests that these foods should replace some of the fatty meats in our diets.[51]

The power of soy lies within powerful compounds known as soy isoflavones. Soybeans contain two major isoflavones: genisten and daidzein. The isoflavones are converted to hormone-like compounds by intestinal bacteria. Other agents found known as saponins have been shown to increase hypocholstrolemic activity, are stimulating to the immune system and antitumoric.

Additionally, clinical trials involving the consumption of isoflavones reveals their ability to help prevent hormone-related cancers. Isoflavones have the ability to stop the uptake of estrogen by estrogen-sensitive tissues.[52] This fact was expressed by Elizabeth Somer, author of *Nutrition For Women,* on the television show Good Morning America. She stated, "that soy products contain substances called phytoestrogens, which mimic the actions of estrogen." Ms. Somer went on to say that studies conducted thus far have revealed that women who consume soy on a regular basis report up to a 40 percent drop in hot flashes, and night sweats.[53]

Recent evidence cited by Dr. Aaron T. Tabor, M.D., Medical Director of Physicians' Laboratories, Winston Salem, NC, reveals that soy has the ability to stop fat cells from storing excess body fat. According to Dr. Tabur, medical researchers at Iowa State University found that soy can:[54]

- decrease the amount of fat your body stores;
- increase your lean muscle mass;
- increase thermogenisis (fatburning) within your fat cells;
- help decrease your appetite; and
- help stabilize blood sugar thus encouraging the body to make energy more efficiently.

The last bullet relates to the Glycemic Index Response to foods. This index is concerned with foods and how fast they raise blood sugar (insulin) levels and is determined by:

- the amount of food you consume;
- how much fat is in it as well as added fat content;
- fiber content.

Lower glycemic foods such as soy sustain energy longer by helping to balance blood sugar levels. As an added benefit, your body will store less fat.

Recent research has shown the health-giving properties of lecithin, a constituent of soybeans, is what biochemists call a phosphatide. A phosphatide is an essential constituent of all living cells, both animal and vegetable. In 1911, in Moscow, Russia, a scientist named Antischkow made the first discovery that later led to the identification of fat as the killer in cases of hardening of the arteries.[55] Researchers have found that lecithin has the ability to increase protective substances that counteract the harmful effects of atherosclerosis from the arteries of experimental animals. Dr. Meyer Friedman, Dr. Sanford Byers and Dr. Ray Rosenman, all of San Francisco, produced fatty plagues in the arteries of experimental animals by feeding large amounts of cholesterol and fats to research animals. Dr. Friedman and his associates concluded from their research that in atherosclerosis, as the fats and cholesterol are removed from the artery walls and flood the blood stream, that the atherosclerotic plagues are dissolved and removed by the lecithin.[56]

While scientists now believe that soybeans and/or soy products have a direct relationship with the reduction of harmful fats, Dr. H. W. Dietrich of Texas maintains that soybeans should be included in the diets of all diabetics. Dr. Dietrich contends that soybeans, essentially, decrease the need for insulin. According to Dr. Dietrich, tests reveal that soybeans lessen the amount of sugar passed in the urine and therefore insulin requirements go down.[57]

Note: *The form of soy that is eaten determines its level of absorption and therefore its nutrient benefit. Unfermented and unsprouted soy (most products) contain an enzyme inhibitor, which limits the body's ability to digest and therefore absorb soy. There is evidence that the need to supplement with the enzyme trypsin is warranted to override the inhibitors when consuming unfermented or unsprouted soy products.*

Spirulina

This one-celled form of algae is known as Nature's wonder food. Because of its ability to synthesize high-quality concentrated food more efficiently than any other algae, it is being developed as the "food of the future." Spirulina is 65 to 71 percent complete protein, with all essential amino acids in perfect balance. In comparison, beef is only 22 percent protein.

Spirulina is characterized by its blue-green color due to its content of chlorophyll and carotenoids (carbon-like pigments, similar in structure to vitamin A). Besides providing a base of solid nutrition, it is viewed as a viable option in the treatment of obesity. Because of its phenylalamine content, it has a controlling effect on hunger as well as the ability to modulate blood sugar. Additionally, due to the actions of chlorophyll, spirulina increases peristaltic action, hastening the removal of waste and undesirable fatty deposits. There is also evidence that spirulina is rich in gamma-linolenic acid (GLA) — the same substance found in evening primrose oil. The gamma linolenic acid content of this oil has a stimulating effect on metabolic cycles.

Moreover, as reported by Dr. Richard Passwater, Director of Nutritional Researcher for Solgar Corp., large-scale clinical trials have substantiated the fact that fatter people tend to have less polyunsaturated fatty acids present. When administered, GLA has been in trials very effective in causing weight loss.[58]

In fact, Dr. K.S. Vaddadi of Bootham Park Hospital in York, England, and Dr. David Horrobin, Medical Director of Efamol Ltd, in the UK found that when test subjects were given evening primrose oil, it lowered body weight in about half of those who were more than 10 percent overweight. This effect was achieved without dieting, although those who lost weight also reported feeling less hungry.[59]

Herbs

Herbs have been used throughout mankind both as medicine and as food. In fact, before the dawn of the "Drug Age," herbs were the mainstay in the treatment of virtually every ailment known to humankind. Today, herbs are still used in the treatment of various diseases within the pharmacological world. However, due to advances in medicine, many herbal preparations are synthetically processed to exceedingly high doses, and as such are used as over-the-counter drugs. Many herbal preparations actually go beyond this level and become the main source of medicine for the primary care needs of possibly 80 percent of the world's population.

Although herbal medicines are widely used and are preferred treatments for many disorders in Europe and Asia, they have not gained wide acceptance in the United States as daily remedies. The following information provides a snapshot of a few of the most popular herbal preparations used today as weight and fat loss aids. In fact, according to a theory known as the "Doctrine of Signatures" the appearance, size or shape of a plant (herb) correlates to and has inherent properties, which are capable of influencing the actions of the internal organ it resembles.

Garlic

Somewhere between folklore, myth, black magic, ancient Chinese and herbal medicine, garlic may finally be getting its due from the medical establishment. Garlic is an herb that has been used for over 4,000 years as a restorer of health, vitality, and as an immune booster. Ancient records dating back as early as 3,000 B.C. show that garlic was used as a medicine by Babylonians, Chinese, Greeks, Romans, Egyptians and Vikings. The great physicians of old, including Galen and Hippocrates (the father of medicine and naturopathy) used garlic to cure everything from intestinal infections and digestive disorders to high blood pressure. During World War II, the Russian and British armies used garlic to control infections in wounds. Garlic was given internally to increase resistance against infections, as well as used externally to speed the healing of the wounds.[60]

A recent article in the Science Times section of the New York Times reported that in laboratory studies and patient trials, garlic preparations had shown the ability to suppress the formation and growth of cancer cells and to counter blood conditions that foster atherosclerosis, heart attacks and strokes. Dr. William J. Bolt of the National Cancer Institute gave praise to these studies and the results of others concerning people in China and Italy. Both studies showed that low rates of stomach cancer were associated with eating a lot of garlic and related vegetables like scallions and onions.[61]

The herb apparently increases the excretion of neutral and acidic sterols, while at the same time suppressing excess cholesterol and lipid (fat) synthesis in the liver. It has also been found that garlic components hold back the production of key enzymes involved in the production of cholesterol and lipids such as hydroxymethyl glutaryl coenzyme A (HMG-CoA) and fatty acid synthetase (FAS). More recent reviews, meta-analyses and epidemiological trials "strongly suggest that garlic (in supplement form) is an effective cholesterol-lowering agent," says Christopher Silagy, Ph.D., and Andrew Neil, M.S.C. in a 1994 article which appeared in Current Opinion in Lipidology.[62] There are compounds in garlic that contain factors which prevent blood clotting and fatty build-up of deposits in arteries, as well as controlling fatty acid oxygenation.[63]

As this ancient seasoning herb begins to gain national attention, enthusiasts are seeking advice concerning its miraculous benefits. Recently, the New York Hospital at Cornell Medical Center announced the opening of its new *Garlic Information Center*, which offers the latest, most up-to-the-minute information concerning research on garlic supplements and the potential benefits of garlic. The center is co-directed by two nationally acclaimed medical and nutrition authorities, Dr. Richard S. Rivlin, M.D., Professor of Medicine at Cornell University Medical College, and Dr. Barbara Levine, Ph.D., R.D., Director for the Nutrition Information Center at Memorial Sloan-Kettering Cancer Center.

Also according to Steven Foster, a world-renowned expert on herbal and botanical substances, garlic has been the subject of intensive research over the past twenty years. In this period, more than 1,000 papers on all aspects of the elementary, pharmacology and clinical uses of garlic have been published. Garlic's benefits can be shown by the following studies.

- Drs. Suzanne G. Yu of the University of Wisconsin at Madison, Dr. Asaf Qureshi of Advanced Medical Research (Madison, WI) and Dr. Robert I. Lin of Nutritional International (Irvine, CA) found that garlic works by blocking the action of the enzyme HMG-COA reductase. Why is this important? This is the same manner in which the popular cholesterol-lowering drugs Lovastatin and Pravastatin work.[64]

- S. Nakagwa and co-workers wrote in the January 1988 issue of Phytotherapy Research that aged garlic extract has shown to protect the liver from the damaging effects of carbon tetrachloride and other potent toxins.

- In a five-month double-blind placebo controlled study by Yeh and associates, as reported in the 1995 Journal of American College Nutrition, aged garlic extract has shown the ability to reduce total plasma and LDL cholesterol by 7 percent and 10 percent respectively. The group studies consisted of free-living males with high cholesterol levels (241 mg LDL) and consuming habitual diets.

- In the 1985 Hiroshima Journal of Medical Science, Nakagaud and fellow researchers revealed that clinical trails show that garlic has the ability to possible reverse damaged liver cells.

- Scientific data has confirmed that garlic effectively reduces blood cholesterol levels in two ways. First, it slows down endogenous (growing or proceeding from within) cholesterol synthesis. Secondly, it helps your body transport fat from tissues where they are stored, to the bloodstream; which enables them to be eliminated from the body.[65]

Cayenne

This herb stimulates peripheral circulation that strengthens the heart and provokes thermogensis (the natural heat process), which accelerates the body's metabolic rate and fatburning capabilities.

Milkthistle

In Germany, this compound is an approved substance in the treatment of alcholism and problems related to faulty liver functions. Milkthistle, which contains *Silymarin,* one of the most powerful flavonoids (an antioxidant), helps liver cells produce glutathione, a liver detoxifier. Since the liver is responsible for the production of bile, which is necessary for the breakdown of fat, we cannot stress too much the importance of this herb and its correlation with proper liver function.

Additionally, part of the silybin molecule is naturally steroidal, assisting in new DNA and ribosomal RNA synthesis. The active agent Silymarin, also causes biomutation of liver cellular membranes to stop the absorption of many toxins. Moreover, milkthistle protects, rejuvenates and prevents fatty accumulation of the liver in a suppression of the diminishing effects of cholangitis (inflammation of bile ducts resulting in decreased bile).

Ginger

Researchers have discovered that ginger inhibits platelet aggregaton (the clumping of blood), which can cause heart attacks, as well as reduce fatty deposits as a result of hypercholesterolemia (excess cholesterol in the blood).[66] When taken hot, ginger produces sweat, thus helping relieve edema and the release of excess toxins. Besides being very effective as an antinauseant in controlling the ill effects of motion sickness, ginger has mild stimulative properties and may help to promote circulation. Studies also suggest that this herb will lower cholesterol.[67]

Yohimbe (Corynanthe Yohimbe)

This herb is very popular and is touted as an aphrodisiac (sexual stimulant). Pure yohimbine has been used by medical professionals to treat male impotence. Researchers contend that it is yohimbe's ability to increase circulation, which is the reason for its commercial appeal to men as a sexual stimulant. Studies have however shown that this herb has the ability to increase fatty acid utilization, preparing stored fat to be used as fuel.[68]

Yohimbine can be purchased over the counter, but has legal limits of up to 3 mg per tablet (this is its purified form). The herbal extract is known as Yohimbe. Yohimbine is thought to have an affect on $alpha_2$ receptors. For women, this poses a unique problem in relationship to lower body fat. Women have many more $alpha_2$ receptors. In fact, there are nine times the number of $alpha_2$ receptors in lower body fat, as compared to $beta_1$ receptors. For this reason Yohimbe would be an excellent fatburning product for women, as well as men.

The $alpha_2$ receptors are believed to have a direct effect with the accumulated storage and proliferation of fat cells (the so-called stubborn lower body fat). This indicates a problem primarily for women, since men have very few $alpha_2$ receptors. According to the late Dan Duchaine, one of the most controversial and prolific writers concerning androgens and their thermogenic effect, when adrenaline or noradrenaline stimulate alpha$_2$ receptors, fat cell mobilization of fatty acids out of the cell is blocked. This inhibition of alpha$_2$ adrenergic receptor sites can be compared to placing tape over a light switch to prevent the lights from being turned on.

Also, at the same time body temperature drops due to noradrenaline generation via nerve endings, thus slowing down the thermogenic process. To make matters worse, low-calorie diets accelerate the production of alpha$_2$ receptors, another major reason why dieting makes you fat. Studies suggest that yohimbine may have some therapeutic effect as an alpha$_2$ blocker.

Note: *Because yohimbe can be classified under the heading of a neuro-hormone, which causes the stimulation of the central nervous system, long-term use is not recommended. Certain other herbal preparations such as kolanut, coffee, tea, guarana and yerbemate also all have traces of the xanthine alkaloids. Xanthines can increase metabolism in the absence of adequate nutritional provisions. As such, many experts do not suggest this mode of action for any substantial amount of time.*

Mahuang

This popular herb also known as ephedra (Ephedra Sinica) has been used for more than 4,000 years to treat asthma and upper respiratory complications. It contains two alkaloids (organic nitrogen containing compounds), ephedrine and pseudoephedrine, which today are found in many popular over the counter cold and allergy medications. Studies conducted to assess the effectiveness of Mahuang's ability, have revealed the fact that it is very effective in reducing lipogenesis (the formation of fat).

Mahuang works by releasing the neurotransmitter in the brain called noradrenaline. When the body pushes adrenalin from the adrenal glands into the blood stream, the brain discharges noradrenaline. This stimulates the body temperature, in effect producing heat, (thermogenesis), thus promoting the breakdown of fat cells. Up to 40 percent of the thermogenic effect of ephedrine is due in part to the activation of Beta-3 receptors. Beta receptors could be compared to a loading dock or refueling station, which interlocks with a truck or an airplane so that refueling can take place. In the human body, these receptors found on fat cells initiate fatburning. When Beta-3 receptors are stimulated by mahuang fatburning activities increase.

When Beta-3 receptors are animated, this causes fat loss without loss of muscle.

To understand the process by which a dynamic cycle of fat burning is ignited, we must first understand how cells operate. The cell itself is a bustling metropolis, each one having its own power plant, its own digestive system, its own factors for making proteins and other molecules. One of the most important elements of a cell's activity is the complex communication network through which it can regulate its own activity. For example, deciding when to reproduce, as well as receive and transmit messages from hormones and or other cells. This intricate process is in part controlled by the protective covering that surrounds the cell called the plasma membrane, which is much like your outer skin that serves as a protective barrier.

According to Daniel Mazia of the University of California, Berkeley, the cell membrane is not a wall, skin or sieve—it is an active and responsive part of the cell. It decides what is inside and what is outside and what the outside does to the inside via small sites located on its surface called receptors.[69]

There are two broad types of receptors (beta and alpha). Ephedine is an alkaloid (active compound) found in Ephedra (mahuang), which is a stimulator of all three subcategories of beta receptors. In the human body, these receptors – found on fat cells – initiate fatburning. When Beta-3 receptors are stimulated by mahuang, fatburning activities increase. $Beta_1$ signals the cell to store fat. $Beta_2$ and $beta_3$ are thermogenic-type receptors which instruct the mitochondria (the power plants of the cells) to burn more fatty acids (fats broken down) to produce heat.

It is here that ephedra (Mahuang), which interacts with receptors on the plasma membranes, initiates its powerful thermongenic (fat-burning) effect. Besides directing the traffic of nutrients, waste and other materials in and out of the cell, the plasma membrane controls the cell's communication system, transmitting signals from its outer environment (including signals from other cells), as well as sending out its own messages. Many of the signals are activated by chemical couriers called hormones. Hormones have general effects throughout the body and initiate specific actions of certain target cells of tissues.

Most hormones stimulate target cells by attaching to predetermined biological sites on the membranes of the cell. Ephedra (Mahuang) stimulates specific receptors initiating its fatburning effect. As hormones reach each target cell, they generally cannot pass through the membrane due to their solubility. They instead trigger intricate responses, giving signals to specific receptors on the cell surface. In turn, these receptors then activate a backup, or second messenger system, which passes along orders for the appropriate changes to occur within the cell.

Ephedra (Mahuang) is a central nervous stimulant and as such is not recommended for those suffering from heart disease, diabetes, thyroid dysfunction or high blood pressure. Recommended dose is 335 to 670 mg of mahuang, which is equivalent to 25 to 50 mg of ephedrine. Do not exceed recommended dose.[70] There are reports that the FDA intends on banning supplements that contain more than 8 milligrams (mg) as well as limiting the maximum dose to 24 mg a day.

It is here that Steven Foster, a well-known botanist of the American Botanical Council in Austin, Texas, contends that ephedra is perhaps the most misunderstood stimulant sold in America. He states that ephedra product labels that list pseudoephedrine or ephedrine among their ingredients may be expected to have a much stronger effect on the body than the dried ephedra herb, which is generally safer when used appropriately.[71] Moreover, Larry Hobbs, author of *Ephedrine and Caffeine: The Ideal Diet Pill*,[72] states that people with "nervous personalities" seem to be more susceptible to side effects from ephedrine. He suggests beginning with smaller than normal amounts and thereafter slowly increasing the dose. This will give the body time to adjust and in many cases reduces any negative side effects.

Note: *On April 17, 2001, Governor Miles Johanns of Nebraska approved legislation that revoked a previous ban on ephedrine and pseudoephedrine products being sold as over-the-counter (OTC) items. Citing abuse or misuse by some users versus potential health problems, these products have been reclassified as OTC items versus prescription drugs.*

It is in this context that Mark Blumenthal, founder and Executive Director of the American Botanical Council, argues that negative press concerning botanicals (herbs) often are slighted, without any benefits discussed concerning the products' efficacy.

St. John's Wort

St. John's Wort's use dates back to the middle ages. Over the years, this herb has been used as a mild tranquilizer and as a treatment for depression and insomnia. A great deal of the recent interest in St. John's Wort was stimulated by a 1994 study which appeared in the Journal of Geriatric Psychiatry and Neurology. This study followed the herb's effects on 3,250 patients suffering most from mild to moderate depression. Results showed up to 80 percent of the participants either felt better or became completely free of symptoms after about four weeks.[73] Additionally, Raymond Reichert in his examination found that St. John's Wort faired better in head to head trails with the antidepressive drugs Maprotiline hydrochloride and Imipramine.[74]

In the above study, 135 patients suffering from depression were administered either 900 mg of St. John's Wort per day, or 75 mg (a day) of imipramine for six weeks. The St. John's Wort-treated group rated better than the imipramine group, as measured by the Hamilton Depression Scale (a standard scale used to determine degree and levels of depression). For those of you who suffer from the depression and anxiety dieting can cause, St. John's Wort may be the ideal mood elevator to compliment the stimulating effect of Mahung.

One of the added benefits of St. John's Wort, according to Dr. Joseph Di Bartolemeo, M.D., the formulator of Herbal Fen-Phen, is its ability to raise serotonin levels, similar to the drug Fen-fluamine.[75] Data has corroborated St. John's Wort's capability of increasing serotonin levels by the synergist effects of St. John's Wort, together with 5-Pyridoxal Phosphate (a form of Vitamin B_6). This combination was found to increase synthesis of serotonin by as much as 60 percent.[76]

St. John's Wort also acts as a mild diuretic and contains 0.1% of the red fluorescent coloring Hypericin and Pseudohypericin. Its effectiveness is attributed to the Hypericin in particular. Recent research from New York Medical University and the Weizman Institute of Science in Israel have found that the two above agents in St. John's Wort can inhibit the growth of the AIDS virus in animals.[77] Trials conducted with St. John's Wort have demonstrated its ability to improve REM sleep, the deepest and most relaxed state of rest. This state is ideal for body repair and fatburning cycles. Data suggests that St. John's Wort can have a tonic effect on the ventricles of the heart, the aorta and arterioles. Minimal dosages have shown the ability to be very effective in increasing blood flow to stressed tissue.

Herbs and the Colon: Dr. Robert H. Sorge, Ph.D., N.D., Director of the Abunda Life Health Hotel and Clinic, in Asbury Park, New Jersey, and author of *"Bowel Management and Colon Irrigation Therapy"*, states that "fat is nothing but the storage of excess metabolic material the body can't process, mainly from the colon."[78] Dr. Sorge goes on to say that for most obese persons, their metabolism can be compared to a car that has eight cylinders; but is only firing on three. This misfiring correlates with slow and sluggish actions of one's automobile, exhibiting no power and or thrust. If the colon is not working correctly, no other organ can function at peak levels; thus causing severe metabolic efficiency.

One of the major problems in the above scenario is with the mal-absorption of fats. When the colon is inundated with hypochondriacal (unhealthy) material, these constituents are dumped into the bloodstream. In turn, as the fire alarm sounds, alternative dumpsites are sought out. This occurrence can be compared to a garbage truck loaded with unwanted material, with no dumpsite available. According to Dr. Sorge, since fat cells of the body are storage cells, they become the primary cites for the depositing of these undigested fats and other by-products of the metabolic process. This perpetual cycle of events is believed to be a key factor in accelerating weight gain, and hindering repeated attempts at reducing fat stores.

Current data suggest that permanent fat loss cannot be truly achieved until the problems associated with improper functioning of the colon are corrected. During this millennium, colon therapy and its application should serve as a practicable option in treating clinical obesity.

To further clarify this point, studies conducted at the National Chiropractic College have shown that the average person is carrying around 20 to 40 pounds of impacted fecal matter in their colons.[79] Additionally, thanks to the pioneering research by the late Bernard Jensen, D.C., world-renowned author, scientist, nutritionalist and researcher, we now know that slow gastrointestinal elimination can have serious consequences. The slower the process, the more difficult and, in some cases, weight and fat loss become impossible.

The following herbal products have a long history of use for their ability to cleanse and purify the colon greatly assisting the body in its ability to metabolize fats and other byproducts of normal metabolism:

•alfalfa, •fennel seeds, •aloe vera, •golden seal root; •bladder wrack; •milkthistle; •black walnut; •Oregon grape root; •senna •burdock root; •peppermint; •butchers broom; •red clove; •capsicum; •reishi; •cascara sagrada; •rhubarb; •chamomile; •dandelion root; •yellow dock.

Hormones

There has been a recent explosion of clinical trials concerning the effects of hormones and the mechanisms they control. Scientists are exploring ways not only to maintain life span, but improve our quality of life. These chemical messengers circulate throughout the body, helping genes turn on in order to regulate the actions of different cells, accelerating their growth, maintaining their structure, function and even how they repair themselves. In essence, hormones are organic molecules secreted in one part of the body and then carried by the bloodstream to other tissues and organs where they exert specific effects. The effects of a hormone on its specific tissue, depends on the presence in the target cells of receptors specific for that hormone.

Many of the mechanisms designed to preserve our existence begin to decline in production as we age. This decline in the output and function of many bodily processes including metabolism and proper fat distribution can be referred to as "the invisible hand of Nature." During this downtime, critical biological processes that are controlled by hormonal actions, begin to slow down. As we learned in previous chapters, there is a dramatic decline in body muscle mass, which is being replaced biologically with fat and flab. The body also tends to increase its production of cholesterol causing the development of fatty deposits that could result in severe health consequences if not controlled.

Researchers have isolated many of these hormonal compounds, which are now used to support the body's natural thermogenic (fat reducing) cycles. Two of these hormonal agents, DHEA and Melatonin, are reviewed below.

DHEA

DHEA stands for dehyroepiandrosterone. DHEA is the most abundant hormone found in the human bloodstream. Production of this hormone begins at the fetus stage, ends at birth, and resumes again around age seven. Researchers believe that DHEA levels begin to decline at age 25. By age 60, its levels have slipped to almost 90 percent from peak output. The adrenal glands and gonads (testes and ovaries) are responsible for releasing DHEA into the circulation.

Recently, DHEA has been the subject of over four thousand scientific studies, and has received national attention from the media for its remarkable ability to halt the aggression of several age-related factors. This hormone has been shown to decrease appetite, stimulate fat metabolism and induce thermogenic activity.

Research has shown that this super hormone has the ability to speed up the rate at which fat and carbohydrates are used. Excess carbohydrates, which are not used as fuel, are consequently stored as body fat. DHEA may actually help create more energy and reduce fat storage. In fact, in a study conducted at the Medical College of Virginia, five normal men were given a placebo and five normal men were given DHEA. In only 20 days, those in the DHEA group saw their mean percent of body fat decrease by 31 percent with no change in weight.[80] Scientists have in their research found that DHEA suppresses appetite (at least in rats) while others demonstrated DHEA's potential to decrease body fat composition and plasma glucose.[81]

The reduction ability of DHEA in reference to plasma glucose (blood sugar) levels is of critical importance in cases of severe obesity. Over time, as glucose seeps through the blood and tissues, it can react with proteins and cause them to permanently link together (known as crosslinking). This will hamper the body's ability to burn stored fats, as well as the proper utilization of carbohydrates due to the excessive glucose. Although glucose is used to fuel many bodily systems, constant over-production may result in stiff-joints, clogged blood vessels and brittle bones.

Natural enhancement of DHEA has been reported to increase with physical exercise, stress reduction programs and transcendental meditation. In fact, studies have shown higher serum DHEA levels in all age groups of women and most age groups of men who practice transcendental meditation regularly. DHEA levels in "meditators" have been shown to be comparable to those of nonmeditators.

Note: A word of caution: *Due to the 1994 Dietary Supplement Health and Education Act (DSHEA) signed into law by President Clinton, DHEA can be purchased over the counter. Drug and vitamin stores usually carry dosages that range from 25 to 50 mg. While short-term studies of DHEA use have yet to show any harmful* *effects, individuals prone to or have problems related to hormonal influences such as breast, ovarian or uterine cancer, prostate problems, and/or liver disease should refrain from using this product, unless specified by their personal physician. DHEA may help to preserve islet cells in the pancreas, which control the release of insulin. When islet cells were exposed to a compound that reduced glucose-sensitive insulin release, the potentiated cells did not return to normal function. But when the same cells were cultured in a laboratory dish with DHEA for up to eighteen hours, insulin release function had been restored. These researchers concluded that DHEA has the ability to reset the inhibitory actions of glucose metabolism and as such have the potential to protect the cells from nitric oxide syntheses and related toxicities.*[82]

Current studies of DHEA sulfate levels have been implicated and correlated with lower levels of obesity in relationship to body fat distribution, as measured by waist/hip ratio in a sample of 151 healthy women aged 18 to 24 years. Scientists suggest that the higher the ratio of DHEA sulfate (into which DHEA is freely converted in the body), the greater the possibility of less body fat and obesity.[83] There is evidence that DHEA supplementation (100 mg) for up to six months can have a dramatic effect on accelerating lean body mass levels in both men and women.[84]

Melatonin

According to recent reports, scientists have unlocked some of the amazing benefits of melatonin. Researchers have found that this substance participates in a variety of critical body processes by:

- setting the body's daily rhythms (such as the onset of sleep);
- treating jet lag;
- fighting depression;
- slowing down the aging process;
- combating cancer;
- stimulating metabolism;
- increasing visual acuity;
- stimulating the release of growth hormone, thus promoting fatburning;
- protecting the body from free radical damage; and
- decreasing cholesterol and excessive fatty deposits.

Melatonin is secreted from the pineal gland; a pea-sized structure nestled at the center of the brain. Melatonin's secretions occur in the absence of light. As night approaches, the pineal gland starts its production of melatonin, which is circulated to all parts of the body. When light hits the retina, neural impulses signal the pineal gland to slow down melatonin production. As this natural phenomenon takes place, our biological clock is being set. Melatonin levels vary on a diurnal basis (from day to night) and on a seasonal basis; for example, when winter days are shorter than summer days.

Circadian biological rhythms play an important part in human functioning and aging. By controlling the action of other hormones, melatonin keeps us in sync with various cycles of body functions, up to and including fat-burning cycles. Melatonin's production is controlled by the enzyme NAT (N-Acety-Transfense). Activation of NAT depends not only as a result of light hitting the retina of the eye; but is activated from information relayed from the brain.

Daylight ➡ Activation of NAT
Food Consumption ➡ Transmutation to Tryptophan
➡ Body converts Tryptophan to Serotonin
Nightfall➡ Serotonin is converted to Melatonin

Researchers have been documenting melatonin's sleep-inducing properties since the early 1980s. It is this resting phase that is crucial to the body's ability to successfully burn excess body fat and tissues during the nocturnal (sleep) process. Finding substances that stimulate the pituitary gland, thus releasing this powerful fat-burning hormone has become commonplace.

One of these, Human Growth Hormone (HGH) enhances immune activity and stimulates growth, sparking institutions such as the National Institute on Aging, to sponsor clinical trails that investigate its influence on body composition. Dr. Daniel Rudman of the Medical College of Wisconsin, reported in 1990 that when elderly men with low levels of growth hormone were given supplements, their fat shrank by 14 percent and their lean body mass expanded by 9 percent.[85]

Melatonin normalizes growth hormone levels, thus stabilizing blood sugar levels. This hormone appears to also regulate the production of corticosteriods (produced as a result of stress), which increase the production of glucose, which raises blood sugar levels, thus provoking an insulin response. This excess response is implicated in accelerating hardening of the arteries due in part to faulty fat metabolism.[86] Due to the fact that muscle is a much more metabolic agent and much healthier in reference to cariovascular health, melatonin's action on its production of growth hormone has been the subject of intense investigation. In other words, melatonin has a positive affect on blood lipids (fat) that clog your arteries by modulating stress reactors in the body that perpetuate the insulin response. It is insulin that encourages the body to store fat. Also, because of melatonin's ability to stimulate growth hormone production, the body is better able to foster lean muscle growth versus fat storage.

Androstenedione

This hormone was made famous by Mark McGuire, the baseball homerun king. It is touted and widely used by bodybuilders because it is a direct precursor to testosterone. The hormone's pre-genenolone and DHEA have three to four different bio-chemical processes before they are converted to testosterone. Androstenedione has only one. Current data indicates that 50 to 100 milligrams can help increase lean muscle gains.[87]

Vitamins and Minerals

As a nutritional consultant, I have found that many people are aware of nutritional benefits from taking vitamin and mineral supplements. In fact, a recent survey conducted by Applied Biometrics located in North Palm Beach, Florida, indicated the number one reason adults took bionutritional substances was to prevent disease. According to Dr. A. Elizabeth Sloan, Ph.D., President of Applied Biometrics, many of the participants of this study (24 percent) said that they purchased supplements to "treat" (as opposed to prevent) medical conditions. Dr. Sloan recommends the opposite position, which is the use of supplements as long-term preventive measures. Categories that looked at weight loss or reducing body fat were not included in this study.

Vitamins and minerals are in many respects nature's biological catalyst. They initiate and control the actions of many of life's processes, up to and including fatburning. Over the past several decades, vitamin supplementation has increased two-fold. Recent survey results have revealed that multivitamin supplements are the most popular.[88] Vitamins are organic (living) substances that are absolutely essential to life in small quantities. They act as co-factors or co-enzymes that help start or initiate an action in many of the body's metabolic processes. Vitamins play a key role in many of the body's biochemical reductional processes. To ensure you are getting the most efficient return from your weight loss/fat program, it may be wise to consider adding a full multivitamin supplement to your daily regimen.

The group of vitamins we will focus our attention on are the B-vitamins, although many more are involved in some capacity with how the body handles fat. Like most things in nature, the B-vitamins do not stand alone. Eleven different B-vitamins have been isolated by scientists. Research has confirmed that over-administration of a single B vitamin can result in clinical signs of deficiency of the others. To assure your safety, health officials recommend taking them as a group commonly called "B-complex." The list below represents a few of the most popular nutritional supplements that can indirectly assist you in reaching your goals.

Vitamin B-1

This B-vitamin, known as thiamine, was popularized between 1920 and 1929 when an average of 17,000 deaths occurred in Japan alone from a disease known as Beriberi, characterized by nervousness, general debility, loss of hearing, weight loss, local paralysis and finally death. We are protected from this malady by B-1.

Current research has shown that thiamin is directly involved with the metabolism of carbohydrates, thus discouraging storage of fat. Additionally, while acting as a powerful antioxidant thiamin (B-1), plays a critical role in reducing the oxidation of fats in the body, which has been implicated with causing hardening of the arteries and accelerating the aging process.

A thiamin deficiency can slow down the utilization of two brain neurotransmitters: acetylcholine and serotonin.[89] These two chemicals have a direct bearing on weight control and nerve impulses. Vitamin B-1 also is intimately involved with the removal of CO_2, or oxidative decarboxylation reactions. The decarboxylation of alpha-keto acids is critical for the transmutation of amino acids (proteins), fat and carbohydrates to fuel. This translates into less storage of fat. Additionally, Vitamin B-1 has shown the ability to enhance food assimilation due to its assistance in manufacturing hydrochloric acid, as well as improving an abnormally low thyroid function. The net result is more efficient metabolism of foodstuffs, a key factor in weight control.

Vitamin B-3

Vitamin B-3 is known as niacin or the anti-pellagra vitamin, because in the early 1900s more than 10,000 people died from Pellagra in the United States. Researchers now know that Niacin is responsible for protecting us against this disease, which also causes paralysis, emotional disturbance and in extreme cases, several mental illness. Further investigations into the efficiency of Niacin has shown Vitamin B-3 to be an effective aid in weight reduction, circulatory disorders, cholesterol and triglyceride disturbances, as well as the ability to potentiate the effect of insulin in glucose metabolism.[90] Niacin bound with chromium (chromium polynicotinate) was found to be more effective when compared with results of other chromium bound supplements tested. Dr. Martin Urberg at Wayne State University in Michigan also has had similar results. In his experiments, participants given chromium and niacin showed improved glucose tolerance to a greater degree than the same doses administered alone.[91]

Niacin was tested on over 8,000 patients in the Coronary Drug Project at the Maryland Medical Research Institute in Baltimore, MD, from 1966 to 1975. Dr. Paul Canner, Ph.D., who headed this study, maintained that niacin was found to be more effective than lipid-lowering drugs like Clofibrate (Altromids) Dextrothyroxine (Choloxin). There is also evidence that niacin has a greater effect on the mechanisms, which keep cholesterol levels on an even keel. When niacin was paired against three grams per day of clofibnate, a cholesterol-lowering drug, niacin was found to be 28 to 48 percent more effective in lowering cholesterol and triglycerides in the blood. Niacin also created a more desirable HDL/LDL ratio.[92] Moreover, researchers at the Cholesterol Research Center, Department of Veteran Affairs Health Care Systems, in Long Beach, California reported in November 2001 that niacin had a profound effect on raising HDL levels, (the good cholesterol) which doesn't clog up the arteries. Physicians at the Beth Israel Hospital in Boston, Massachusetts, gave niacin in daily doses of two thousand milligrams and found that it offered more fat-lowering benefits than traditional medicines.[93] (The RDA for niacin is 19 milligrams for men and 15 milligrams for women.)

Note: *Because niacin dilates blood vessels, it may cause flushing and body itching with the face turning red and a sensation similar to hot flashes. These occurrences are temporary and are not harmful. This flushing can be minimized by taking niacin with a full* *meal and by using a specialized form called inositol hexanicotinate, which doesn't give you the flushing. This form of niacin has been used extensively in Europe to alleviate the symptoms of Raynaud's Disease, which is caused by abnormal spasms of the blood vessels in a person's extremities.*

The bottom line is that niacin will improve your circulation, thus cleaning and clearing your bloodstream and veins of unwanted accumulation of fats, as well as their utilization for fuel.

Vitamin B-6

Vitamin B-6 is chemically known as Pyridoxine, Pyridoxal, and Pyridoxamine. In its active form, Pyridoxal Phosphate acts as a coenzyme in the metabolism of fats, proteins and carbohydrates. In carbohydrate transformations, the coenzyme works with phosphorylase (a phosphate molecule) which helps convert glycogen (stored blood sugar) to glucose for conversion to energy. Without B-6, this conversion would not take place.

Current scientific information suggests an adjustment in B-6 intake in relationship to protein intake for proper metabolism, muscle growth and stable blood sugar levels. For example, if you are consuming 150 grams of protein, you should take 15 mg of B-6 per day.[94] Vitamin B-6 acts as a shuttle bus transporting amino acids (the end product of protein digestion) across the mucusal wall and into the cell, where they are metabolized.

Current data also has validated Vitamin B-6's role as a valuable tool in weight reduction due to its ability to alleviate edema (water retention). Dr. John M. Ellis, M.D., of Texas, maintains that Vitamin B-6 sets up a balance of the minerals, sodium and potassium. This eliminates the possible use of dangerous diuretics, which can create other complications due to the loss of valuable electrolytes.[95] Vitamin B-6 actually creates an environment for the efficient burning (metabolizing) of fat, carbohydrates and proteins. Additionally, Vitamin B-6 plays an essential role in erythropoiesis and hematopoiesis (the production and development of red blood cells) therefore building the very fluid responsible for the transport of nutrients and oxygen to cells for energy, an added plus.

Concurrent research has revealed that, besides aiding in the conversion of Trytophan (a brain chemical) to niacin, B-6 is additionally involved with the formation of an enzyme called N-Acetyl-Transfense (NAT), implicated in serotonin production. As we learned in earlier chapters, serotonin is responsible for helping us stay calm and collective, as well as curbing our appetite thus reducing cravings for food. This vitamin is also widely used by women, for a number of reasons related to PMS (Pre-menstrual Syndrome). Due to the work of Dr. Karl Folkers, of the University of Texas, Vitamin B-6 is now an accepted treatment for Carpal Tunnel Syndrome which results in numbness, tingling, pain and stiffness in fingers and hands. The RDA for Pyridoxine is 1.6 to 2.0 mg daily.

Choline and Inositol

These two substances, by many standards, do not fit the description of a vitamin. They are, however, members of the B-vitamin family. The name choline is derived from the Greek word "choler" which means "bile" from which choline was first isolated. Albert E. Holland, Jr., author of *The Importance of Creative Nutrition*, describes this vitamin-like substance by using the word "detergent."[96] He maintains that choline is important in human nutrition for its ability to dissolve the cholesterol and fatty deposits in certain parts of the body. Because choline is a fat and cholesterol emulsifier, its technical name is lipotropic.[97] Choline also plays a critical role in the transport of fat in the bloodstream and their consequent metabolism.

Data has also shown that choline is necessary for the body's ability to make acetylcholine, a key neurotransmitter. Dr. Robert Haas, author of *Eat Smart, Think Smart*, maintains that acetylcholine is the most abundant neurotransmitter in the body. Neurotransmitters are the body's brain chemicals that allow you to think, feel, perform and look your best. These brain chemicals control intelligence, memory, sexuality, sleep, mood and weight loss.

Presently, there is no known daily requirement for choline and although there are no known toxicity levels for choline, officials do not recommend exceeding 1,000 mg daily. For optimal health 25 to 300 milligrams a day is suggested.[98]

Inositol is very closely associated with the functions of choline. These two substances are often used in combination to assist in moving fat from the liver to the cells. Inositol's function is similar to that of choline. Without optimal amounts of these substances, cirrhosis and fatty degeneration of the liver can occur leading to hardening of the arteries.[99] This occurrence can have a devastating effect on your weight- and fat-loss goals, not to mention serious circulatory and cardiovascular problems.

The daily optimal dosage range for inositol is the same as choline. To assess the overall efficiency of these substances several controlled studies have validated their ability to manipulate the control mechanism that encourage proper metabolism of fat.

- Butterworth and Krumdiek, researchers in the Nutrition Program of the School of Medicine of the University of Alabama in Birmingham report that the body requires an enzyme, lecithin cholesterol acyltransferase (LCAT) in order to control the buildup of cholesterol and fatty deposits on the walls of the arteries. These researchers concluded that in order for the body to make self-protecting LCAT, it requires choline.
- Nine men and nine women with high triglycerides and cholesterol were given lecithin. Triglycerides, cholesterol and platelet aggregation were significantly reduced, and HDL (the good) cholesterol was increased. The authors concluded that lecithin might be a useful adjunct in the treatment of atherosclerosis.[100]

Note: *As a point of reference, choline and inositol naturally occur in abundance in Lecithin.*

Minerals

Minerals initiate the actions of vitamins, hence the phrase "vitamins are worthless without a full complement of minerals." Moreover, minerals enable proteins to be broken down (for muscle-building) into their component parts (amino acids), making them bioavailable to the body. These substances are vital also to proper glucose metabolism, as well as a host of other enzyme function that are linked to appetite control, proper metabolism, and the breakdown of fats. It is important to remember that minerals often work synergistically and never act alone. For example, zinc is vital to chromium's function, and must be present in adequate quantities for the passage of glucose (blood sugar) from the bloodstream into the cells. The catalytic action of chromium, a gateway that opens for the proper metabolism of glucose, will not occur without zinc acting as a co-factor or enzyme (partner). Zinc also needs help to function and does so more efficiently when copper is present.

For best results, take a full vitamin and mineral supplement. According to Dr. Roger J. Williams, a world-renowned nutritional researcher, "vitamins and minerals work as a team for best results, either for prevention or for treatment."[101]

Chromium (Picolinate)

Discovered by Dr. Gary Evans, Professor of Chemistry at Bemidji State University in Minnesota, chromium picolinate is the trace mineral chromium bound to picolinic acid, a natural chelator agent used by the body to transport nutrients into the cell. In the case of chromium picolinate, the target agent is insulin. Insulin is critical for the proper metabolism of fat, carbohydrates and protein. Without chromium, insulin cannot do its job properly

Chromium's role, and its interaction with insulin had been substantiated via early research by Dr. Walter Metz, former chief of biological chemistry at the Walter Reed Army Institute of Research, who actually discovered the link between chromium and its reaction with receptor sites (junctions or intermediate pathways) on cell membranes.[102] Consequent experiments validated chromium's ability to reduce harmful cholesterol and triglyceride levels in diabetic and chromium deficient animals.

Today, evidence continues to mount as to chromium picolinate's ability to accelerate fat loss while helping to preserve or even increase lean muscle. As stated, the picolinate form has been found to be much more bioavailable to cells. Recent studies conducted by Deborah Hasten, an exercise physiologist at Louisiana State University, although preliminary at the time (1990), showed a meaningful increase in lean body mass in a beginning weight-training program over a twelve-week period.[103]

Chromium picolinate has shown an ability to lower blood levels of fat and raise HDL (the good) cholesterol in relationship to LDL (the bad) cholesterol. Additionally, researchers have found that chromium picolinate has the ability to lower or stabilize glucose (blood sugar) in humans. Based on these factors, scientists contend that it is a very effective supplement in controlling lipid (fat) disorders.

Furthermore, in a double-blind study conducted on off-season football players given 1.6 milligrams of chromium picolinate over a six-week weight training program, with results revealing that chromium picolinate more than doubled the development of lean body mass. Researchers in this study concluded that the net benefit of adding chromium picolinate was 2 to 1 in terms of just exercise alone.[104]

Chromium is probably one of the most widely used mineral supplements to help fight the battle of the bulge. When biological chromium is present, the body is better able to metabolize fat, curb appetite, maintain energy levels and increase the transportation of amino acids (protein) into muscle cells. The Food and Drug Administration (FDA) recommends taking 50 to 200 mcg/per day of chromium.

Note: *Some researchers claim that chromium picolinate is poorly absorbed by the body. They state that chromium polynicotinate, an alternate form of chromium, may be more effective.*[105]

Iodine

There are a multitude of factors that affect the body's metabolic rate. Your body's metabolic rate determines how well or how fast you are converting the calories that you consume into usable fuel. This process has a tremendous effect on the outcome of your weight-loss and fat-reduction goals. The tiny gland located just below the larynx (your voicebox) in the throat is responsible for regulating your body's metabolic rate.

Dr. Raphael Kellerman, M.D., an internist and medical director of the Life Center in New York City, states that "the thyroid gland, especially an underactive, one can often be the cause of chronic fatigue and weight gain. Undetected, this malady could lead to premature stroke."[106]

The precise mechanism by which the thyroid hormone (called T_3 Triiodothyronine and T_4 Thyroxine) affects the cells is still under investigation. Scientists however do know that these secretions have a direct effect on and increase the number of cellular enzymes which explains their role in metabolism and the fat-burning process. In fact, thyroid hormone secreted in very large amounts, can increase the metabolic rate by as much as 200 percent of normal activity. This is known scientifically as hyperthyroidism. On the other hand, an underactive thyroid (hypothyrodism) can cause a decrease in the metabolic rate up to 50 percent of normal output.

Past and current data have confirmed that the mineral iodine plays a key role in the regulation and stabilization of thyroid functions. In many parts of the world where there are insufficient amounts of iodine in the soil, enlarged goiters are prevalent. The mishap is characterized by an enlargement of the throat area due to the thyroid glands attempt to secret thyroxine. When iodine is lacking, no matter how hard the gland works, its hormones can't be made and/or secreted. Researchers have confirmed that a severe iodine deficiency will eventually cause hypothyrodism. This is the reason that some time ago, government officials ordered iodine to be added to our common table salt. The National Research Council of the U.S., recommends a daily intake of 150 micrograms for men and 150 micrograms for women. The herb kelp is a very popular source of natural iodine.

Note: *Iodine in its medical form is very dangerous and is not meant for internal use. Iodine occurs naturally in food or water and has no toxicity. While iodine has long-range implications for sound thyroid function, if you suspect you have a thyroid problem, a simple blood test can tell you for sure. Check with your health care professional.*

Potassium

Potassium is one of our most important minerals. Its actions, along with sodium, known as the sodium-potassium pump is responsible for cell integrity and life's process. Malfunction of this action can accelerate the negative actions of disease states and a severe breakdown of its actions will result in death. Investigations into this dynamic action between sodium and potassium has revealed that the interior of the cells found in higher animals needs to be high in potassium and low in sodium. The exact opposite is necessary in bodily fluids and blood, with sodium being high and potassium low.

The major functions of potassium in the body are varied, but several key actions have a positive effect in relationship to weight management, which include:

• maintaining proper water balance to prevent water retention, and allow food particles to flow into the cells, thus producing energy;

• stimulates glycogen formation and glucose metabolism to increase the body's ability to metabolize protein for building muscle, as well as increase carbohydrate metabolism. This action will deter fat storage.[107]

In addition, researchers claim that increasing the potassium to sodium ratio will help overweight individuals, those who are hypertensive (high blood pressure) and some diabetics. To augment the action of these two minerals, current data suggests increasing potassium and decreasing sodium. There currently is no recommended dietary allowance (RDA) for potassium. Authors of

The Real Vitamin and Mineral Book, suggest taking 99 to 300 mg for optimal results.

Zinc

This mineral is probably one of the most well-known and commercially used minerals besides calcium. Zinc is a powerful antioxidant and is vital for proper immune system functions, as well as an aid to speeding up the healing time of wounds. It is commonplace to utilize zinc, before and after surgical procedures. Also, zinc is vital to maintain a healthy prostate. It is thought to regulate the metabolism of testosterone (a male hormone) in the prostate gland. Excess testosterone has been implicated as a possible cause of prostate cancer.

In addition to the above, zinc is involved in over 100 enzymatic actions including insulin activity (utilization and breakdown of fat) protein metabolism (for building muscle) and in electron transport for energy production. There is strong evidence to support the connection between low levels of zinc and anorexia nervosa, a problematic abnormal eating disorder. Furthermore, current data suggest that atherosclerosis, (hardening or clogging of the arteries) is caused or initiated by a vessel wall injury or malfunction. A low concentration of zinc may be involved in the initiation of the injury and in inadequate tissue repair, thus accelerating atheroselerosis. Zinc is instrumental in slowing down or reducing fat deposits and other debris, which can clog or build up on artery walls.

---

[1] Clouatre, D., *Anti-fat Nutrients,* Pax Publishing, San Francisco, CA, 1997.

[2] *The 1996, Natural Health Handbook,* Natural Health, Brookline Village, MA, 1996, p. 50.

[3] Apovian, C.M., "The Use of Pharmacologic Agents In the Treatment of The Obese Patient," The Journal of The American Osteopathic Association, Vol. 99, No. 10 Part 2, October, 1999, p.52-55.

[4] www.worldimagenaturals.com, Perfect W-eight, North Plains, OR

[5] "Forget Fat Forever," Virtual Muscle Research Network, NY, Vol. 1, Issue 2, 1997.

[6] West, D.B., Delany, J.P., Carnet, P.M., et.al. "Effects and Energy Metabolism in the Mouse", American Journal of Physiology, 1998; 275; R667-672.

[7] Pearson, D., Shaw, S., *Life Extension A Practical Scientific Approach*, Warner Books, NY, 1982.

[8] Van Gaal, et al., "Exploratory Study of Coenzyme Q10 in Obesity," Folkers and Yamura, Vol 4, 1984, p. 369-373.

[9] Stanko, R. T., et al., "Reduction Of Carcass Fat In Swine With Dietary Addition Of Pihydroxyacetone And Pyruvate." Journal of Animal Science: 67: 1272-1278, 1989.

[10] Marshall, W.J., Clinical Chemistry,: J.B. Luppincott, Phila. PA, 1988.

[11] Hultman, T., et al., "Muscle Creatine Loading In Man", Journal of Applied Physiology, 81 (1996): 232-237.

[12] Hill, H. E., *Introduction To Lecithin*, Pyramid Publications, NY, 1972.

[13] Mindell, E., *Vitamin Bible*, Warner Books, New York, NY, 1991.

[14] Darden, E., *How To Lose Fat*, Anna Publishing Inc., Ocoee, FL, 1977.

[15] Nettl, F., *How To Do Your Protein Arithmetic*, Xipe Press, LaCosta, CA, 1995.

[16] Ibid.

[17] Frenkel, R., et.al, *Carnitive Biosynthesis Metabolism, and Functions*, Academic Press, NY, 1980.

[18] Bland, J. *Medical Applications of Clinical Nutrition*, Keats Publishing, New Cannan, CT, 1983, p. 111.

[19] Lee, W. L., *Amazing Amino Acids*, Keats Publishing, New Canaan, CT, 1984.

[20] Pearson, D., Shaw, S., *The Life Extension Weight Loss Program*, Doubleday and Co., Garden City, NY, 1986, p.334.

[21] Mayer, J., *Human Nutrition*, Charles C. Thomas, Springfield, IL, 1974.

[22] Pearson, D., Shaw, S., *The Life Extension Weight Loss Program*, Doubleday and Co., Garden City NY, 1986, p.67.

[23] Beattie, S. Romano, J., "The 10 Best Performance Supplements", Muscular Development, Ronkonkoma, NY, 1995, 6:50-51.

[24] Mourier, A. et al., "Combined Effect Of Caloric Restriction And Branch Chain Amino Acids Supplementation On Body Composition And Exercise Performance In Elite Wrestlers." International Journal of Sport's Medicine, 1997: 1847-55.

[25] Wurtman, J. J., *The Serotonin Solution*, Random House, NY, 1996.

[26] Schechter, S., Griffonia and 5-HTP, For Your Health, Encinitas CA, Vol 1, Issue 5, Aug. 1997, p.1.

[27] Kramen, P. D., *Listening to Prozac*, Viking Press, NY, 1993.

[28] Bel, N., Artigas, F., "Reduction of Serotonergie Function In Rat Brain By Trytophan Depletion: Effects In Control and Fluvoxamine-Treated Rats", Journal of Neurochemistry, 1996: 67:669-676.

[29] Bio-Medical Tidbits, "5-HTP and Trytophan Dependency," Life Enhancement News, 1996, p. 20.

[30] Wade, C., *Helping Your Health With Enzymes*, Parker Publishing Co., West Nyack, NY, 1966.

[31] Welner, M., "More Precious Than Gold: Enzymes," Gere Vita Laboratories, Toronto, Ontario, Canada, 1997, p.3.

[32] Campbell, R. A., *Biology 3rd Edition*, Benjamin Cummings, Redwood City, CA, 1993, p. 273.

[33] Welner, M., "More Precious Than Gold: Enzymes," Gere Vita Laboratories, Toronto, Ontario, Canada, 1997, p.3.

[34] Howell, E., *Enzyme Nutrition: The Food Enzyme Concept*, Avery Publishing, Garden City Park, NY, 1985.

[35] Welner, M., "More Precious Than Gold: Enzymes," Gere Vita Laboratories, Toronto, Ontario, Canada, 1997, p.3.

[36] Graham, D.Y., "Enzyme replacement therapy of exocrine prancreatic insufficiency in man, relations between invitro enzyme activities and invivo potency in commercial pancreatic extracts." New England Journal of Medicine, 1977: (296): 1314-1317.

[37] Bieler, H. G., *Food Is Your Best Medicine*, Random House, NY, 1965.

[38] Schwartz, R., Ravussin, E., Massari, M., et.al., "The Thermic Effect of Carbohydrate Versus Fat Feeding in Man", Metabolism, Vol. 34 1985: (3): 285-292.

[39] Schlosberg, S., "Food Phobias," *Shape Magazine,* Woodland Hills, CA, March 1998, p.86, p.86-89-139.

[40] Sheats, C., Robinson, M.G., Lean Bodies, Warner Books, NY, 1995.

[41] Anderson, J. W., "Hypercholesterolemic Effects of High - Fiber Diets Rich In Water-soluble Plant Fibers"; Journal of Canadian Diet Association, 1984; 45:140.

[42] Kaneuchi, O., Deuchi, K., Imasato, Y., Shizukuishi, M., Kobayashi, E., "Mechanism For The Inhibition of Fat Digestion By Chitosan and For The Synergistic Effect of Ascorbates, Biosel", Biotechnol., Biochemistry, 5:95; (5): 786-90.

[43] Vahouny, G., Kritchevsky, D.,"Dietary Fiber," Health and Disease, Plenum Press, NY, 1982.

[44] Goodhart, R., Shils, M., *Modern Nutrition In Health and Disease,* Lea and Febiger, Philadelphia, PA, 1980.

[45] Airola, Paavo., N.D., Ph.D., Are You Confused, Health Plus, Phoenix, AZ, 1986.

[46] Burroughs, A., *The Master Cleaner*, Burroughs Books, Auburn, CA, 1993.

[47] Ibid.

[48] Schechter, S., Griffonia and 5 HTP, For Your Health, Encinitas CA., Vol 1. Issue 5, Aug. 1997, p. 2.

[49] Adams, R., Murray, F., *All You Should Know About Health Foods*, Larchmont Books, NY, 1975.

[50] Ibid.

[51] Hausman, P., Foods that Fight Cancer, Rawson Associates, NY, 1983.

[52] Steinberg, P. N., *Isoflavones and the Concentrated Soy Supplements*, Healing Wisdom Publishing, NY, 1996, p. 5.

[53] Mori-Nu, Nutofu "A Delicious Way To Increase One's Intake of Soy, Morinaga" Nutritional Foods, Inc., Torrance, CA, Oct/Nov, 1996.

[54] http://www.doctors@revivalsoy.com. for information on the study and newslettter.

[55] Morrison, L., *Dr. Morrison's Heart-Saver Program*, St. Martin's Press, NY, 1982.

[56] Ibid.

[57] Hill, H. E., *Introduction To Lecithin*, Pyramid Publications, NY, 1972.

[58] Passwater, R.A., Evening Primrose Oil, Keats Publishing Inc., New Canaan CT, 1981, p. 17.

[59] Vaddadi K.S., Horrobin, D.F., "Weight loss produced by evening primrose oil administration in normal and schizophrenic individuals," IRCS Journal of Medical Science 7 (1979): p. 52

[60] Brody, Jane, "Article Reprint", *Science Times (of the New York Times).* September 4, 1990.

[61] Ibid.

[62] Gormely, J. (Ed.), "Garlic, Ancient Wisdom for Today's Healing," Better Nutrition, Atlanta, GA, Oct. 1995, p. 16.

[63] Fogarty, M. "Garlic's Potential Role in Reducing Heart Disease," British Journal of Clinical Practice, 1993, 47 (2): 64-65.

[64] Robert I. Lin, Garlic and Health, International Academy of Health and Fitness, Irvine, CA, 1994, p.7

[65] Mindell, E., Dr. Earl Mindell's Garlic, The Miracle Nutrient, Keats Publishing, New Canaan, CT, 1994.

[66] Foster, S. 101 Medicinal Herbs, Interweave Press, Loveland, CO, 1998, p.99.

[67] Macolo, N., et al., "Enthnopharmalogic Investigation of Ginger (Zingiber Officinale)," Journal of Ethnopharmocelogy, 1989, 27:129-140.

[68] Berlan, M., et al., "Plasma Catecholamire Levels and Lipid Mobilization Induced by Yohimbine in Obese and Non-obese Women," International Journal of Obesity, 15.5: 305-315,1991.

[69] Pines, M., Inside The Cell: The New Frontier of Medical Science, US Department of Public Health, Education and Welfare, Washington DC, 1978, p.66.

[70] Aceto. C., "Eating To Lose," Muscle and Fitness, Woodland Hills CA; March, 1998, p. 93.

[71] Foster, S., "The Misunderstood Herb", Herbs For Health, Vol. 9 Number 2, Dec. 1996/Jan. 1997, p. 66.

[72] Hobbs, L., *Ephedrine and Caffeine: The Ideal Diet Pill*, Pragmatic Press, Irvine, CA, 1996.

[73] Miller, S., "A Natural Mood Booster," Newsweek, May 5, 1997.

[74] Reichert, R., "St. John's Wort Extract As A Tricyclic Medication Substitute For Mild To Moderate Depression", Quarterly Review Nat. Medicine, 1995: 275-278.

[75] Hobbs, L. S., "Rating The Latest Weight Loss Supplements, All Natural Muscular Development", 10:97: 150 (210-212-218).

[76] Hartvig, P., Lindrer, K. J., Byurling, P., Lansotrom, B., Tedroff, J., Pyridoxine "Effect on Synthesis Rate of Serotonin In The Monkey Brain Measured With Positron Emission Tomography," Neural Tran., 1995; 102:91-97.

[77] Mindell, E., *Earl Mindell's Herb Bible*, Simon and Schuster, NY, 1992.

[78] Sorge, R., *The World's Greatest Body-Fat Loss Program,* Abunda Life Holistic Healing Retreat, Asbury Park New Jersey, 1990.

[79] Ibid.

[80] Virtual Muscle Research Network, "Forget Fat Forever," Vol. One, Issue Two, NY, 1997, p.8.

[81] Diamond, P., et al., "Metabolic Effects of 12-month Percutaneous Dehydroeplandrosterone Replacement Therapy in Postmenopausal Women", Journal of Endrocrinology, 1996, 150 Supp. 1): S43-S50.

[82] Laycheck, S. G., Bauer, A. L., "Epiandrosterone and Dehydroeplandrosterone Affect Glucose Oxidation and Interleukin-1 Beta Effects in Pancreatic Islets." Endocrinology, 1996, 137: 3375-3385.

[83] Mantzoros, et. al., "Dehydroeplandrosterone Sulfate and Testosterone and Independently Associated with Body Fat Distribution In Premenopausal Women." Epidemiology, 1996, 7:513-516.

[84] Morales, A. J., et al., "The Yen Study, Effects of Replacement Dose of Dehydroepiandrosterone in Men and Women of Advancing Age," Journal of Clinical Endrocrinological Metabolism, 1994; 78:1360-1367.

[85] Schmidt, "Old No More", Science and Society, U.S. News and World Report, March 8, 1993.

[86] Touitou, Y., Bogdan, A., Auzeby, A., "Activity of Melatonin and Other Pineal Indoles on the InVitro Synthesis of Cortisol, Cortisone and Adrenal Androgens, Journal of Pineal Research, 1989, 6:341-50.

[87] Virtual Muscle Research Network, "Forget Fat Forever," Vol. 1, Issue 2, NY, 1997, p.8.

[88] Council For Responsible Nutrition, Washington, DC, May, 1993.

[89] Liberman, S., Bruning, *Design Your Own Vitamin and Mineral Program,* Double Day, Garden City, NY, 1987, p. 76.

[90] Bland, J. et al., "The Effect of Chromium As Cr (III) Chloride, Yeast Bound Chromium and A Nicotinato Cr (III) Complex On Tissue Uptake, Glucose Tolerance Serum Lipids and et al Development In Rats," Linus Pauling Inst. Of Science and Medicine, Palo Alto, CA, 1986.

[91] Urberg, M., Zemel, M. B., "Evidence For Synergism Between Chromium and Nicotinic Acid In The Control of Glucose Tolerance In Elderly Humans", Metabolism, 36 (9): 896-899, 1987.

[92] Vaugh, L., *The Complete Book of Vitamins and Minerals,* Rodale Press, Emmaus, PA, 1988, p. 94.

[93] Adams, R., *The Big Family Guide To All Vitamins,* Keats Publishing, New Canaan CT, 1992, p. 125.

[94] Phillips, B., *Sports Supplement Review, 3rd Ed.*, Mile High Publishing, Golden, CO, 1997.

[95] Clark, L., *Know Your Nutrition,* Keats Publishing, New Canaan, CT, 1973.

[96] Holland, Albert E., Jr, *The Importance of Creative Nutrition,* Ectolyte, Garden Grove, CA, 1971.

[97] Clark, L., *Know Your Nutrition,* Keats Publishing, New Canaan, CT, 1973.

[98] Liberman, S., Bruning, N., The Real Vitamin and Mineral Book, Avery Publishing, Garden City Park, NY, 1990, p.272.

[99] Hoffer, A., Walker, A., Ortho-molecular Nutrition, Keats Publishing, New Canaan, CT, 1973.

[100] Ibid.

[101] Williams, R., *Nutrition Against Disease*, Pitman Publishing, New York, NY, 1971.

[102] Mertz, W., "Chromium occurrence and function in biological systems," Physiological Review 49, (1969): 163.

[103] DiSpaltro, D., "Chromium Picolinate Scores again in New Fat Reducing and Muscle" Building Study, Nutrition 21, San Diego CA., Aug 31st, 1990.

[104] Evans, G.W., "The effect of chromium Picolinate on insulin controlled parameters in humans," International Journal of Biosocial and Medical Research, 1989.

[105] www.worldimagenaturals.com, Perfect W-eight, North Plains, OR

[106] Kellerman, R., "Energizing Chronic Fatigue", Alternative Medicine Digest, Tiburon, CA, 9:97:60.

[107] Pike, R., Brown, M. L., *Nutrition: An Integrated Approach,* MacMillian Publishing, New York, NY, 1984, p. 177.

Chapter Seven

Natural Diet Aids

In this section, you will find some products that have a large following and are very popular throughout various parts of the world and/or their native country. These products are moving into mainstream America and are gaining notoriety. Additionally, you will find listed a few of the most popular natural fatburners used in the United States.

Note: *Products listed here are not meant to imply any endorsement or preference toward usage by the author. They are listed for information purposes only.*

Garcinia Cambogia: Nature's Natural Fat Buster

While many of us seek out new diets and reduce our calorie intake, a little-known Indian herb is gaining national prominence for its ability in promoting the body's natural fat-burning mechanisms. To date, more than 70 scientific trials have been conducted concerning its safety and effectiveness. The name of this remarkable herb is Garcinia Cambogia. Derived from a native Asian fruit-bearing plant, this all-natural herb decreases appetite, may speed up calorie burning, and inhibits the body's ability to store fat.[1] This orange, pumpkin-shaped fruit (also known as "Malabar tamarind" or "goraka") has been used for years in Thai and Indian cuisines.

Current interest in Garcinia Cambogia stems from the content of hydroxycitric (a component of hydroxycitric acid) found in fruit rinds. The rind (called pericarp) is dried and extracted to produce (-) hydroxycitric acid (HCA). HCA is a close relative to citric acid, which gives oranges, lemons and limes their citrus flavor.

For centuries, people in southern India have used the rind as a natural food preservative, flavoring agent and digestive aid. The (-) form of HCA (referring to the manner in which the molecule is structured) is the naturally occurring form of HCA that exhibits its unique properties. In addition, studies show that HCA is as safe, perhaps safer, than citric acid, which is used extensively in commercial food productions.[2]

In 1965, the active principle in the pericarp of Garcinia Cambogia, initially misidentified as citric acid, was shown to be (-) hydroxycitric acid. Three years later, John M. Lowenstein found that this compound strongly inhibited fatty acid synthesis in living systems.[3] The next year, in an article written in the Archives of Biochemistry and Biophysics, Ann Sullivan reported that fatty acid and cholesterol synthesis were blocked significantly in test animals given (-) hydroxycitrate before being fed.[4] In another journal, Lipids, Ms. Sullivan and her colleagues noted that rats fed (-) hydroxycitrate tended to eat less than did the control animals in the study.[5] They also reported that (-) hydroxycitrate lowered body fat levels with no loss of body protein or lean mass, in test animals that had been experimentally made obese. Based on these dramatic observations, medical scientists began escalating their research on this unique molecule derived from the Malabar Tamarind. In a 1987 study of obese men, a dose of 800 mg per day in a 220-pound person resulted in an average loss of three-and-a-half pounds after only one week.[6]

In 1991, an eight-week, double-blind study was done using 54 volunteers. The 22 subjects in the test group who used Lipodex-2 (a supplement containing 500 mg of Garcinia Cambogia extract and an amino acid chelate of chromium and niacin) lost an average 11.1 pounds per person.[7]

In 1994, an eight-week study was conducted using seventy-five volunteers taking Citrin 75 (a supplement consisting of 250 mg (-) hydroxycitrate and 100 mcg chromium from chromium picolinate). The study group included 60 women and 15 men who ranged in age from 21 to 65 years, and in weight from 135.5 to 253 pounds. Forty-two subjects who completed the study lost an average of 10.8 pounds each.[8]

HCA is not new to the scientific world. Researchers at Brandeis University, Waltham, Massachusetts, published articles on HCA as long ago as 1970, and scientific teams from the pharmaceutical giant, Hoffman-LaRoche, spent two decades exploring the benefits of HCA through animal trials. To date, more than 70 scientific papers have been published which involve research on HCA. Additionally, human trials at the University of Arizona and in Hilton Head, South Carolina showed no side effects. And, of course, there is the record of centuries of use in southern Asia.

Garcinia cambogia is different from other so-called fat-busting pills. When foods are eaten, carbohydrates are digested and broken down into glucose. Glucose is the special blood sugar the body uses for energy. Those foods that are not immediately used for energy are stored in the body's liver and muscles as glycogen. When glycogen stores become full, monitors in the liver called glucoreceptors, send a satiety signal to your brain indicating you are full. When glycogen is not produced or stored in sufficient quantities, more carbohydrate calories are converted into fatty acids (such as triglycerides), or used to produce cholesterol.

The conversion process of carbohydrates into triglycerides and cholesterol requires an enzyme called ATP-citratelyase. HCA works by temporarily inhibiting the action of this enzyme. This is the key to blocking fat production. Benefits revealed studies have shown that HCA controls a dieter's appetite, increases energy levels, maintains blood sugar levels, controls cholesterol and triglyceride levels and may increase thermogenesis (calorie-burning).

Most appetite suppressants act by stimulating the body's central nervous system (CNS). This frequently leads to side effects such as insomnia, nervousness, depression, hypertension and rapid heart rate. The body also tends to develop a tolerance against CNS stimulants, eventually rendering them ineffective. HCA is not a CNS stimulant and won't cause side effects or lead to intolerance by the body. HCA suppresses appetite safely and effectively by working with the body's own natural processes. In fact, according to Dr. Dallas Clouatre, of the University of California Berkley, dieters using adequate amounts of HCA will find a moderate but steady loss of pounds without the usual weight loss roller coaster symptoms. These include the sudden loss of water weight followed by decreased energy and then a dieting plateau, as found with the crash and fad diets.[9]

Research trials suggest that for maximum results, an average-sized person should use from three to six grams of actual HCA, which is six to 12 grams of the highest quality extract. However, based on the clinical studies when HCA was combined with niacin-bound chromium, and when a low-fat/low-sugar/high-fiber diet was followed, a much lower dose was needed.[10] Current data indicates that taking a combination of 250mg HCA plus 100mcg of chromium three times a day will work well for the vast majority of dieters. The active ingredient in garcinia cambogia, HCA, in extensive trials show that HCA should be taken 30 to 60 minutes before meals to be effective, although it can remain active for several hours afterwards. Investigations also show that HCA is 700 percent more effective when taken two times per day rather than when taken only once. Based on this data, researchers suggest that three times per day may even be better.

Rhodiola Rosea and Rhodoendron Caucasicum

In the United States, much of what is considered alternative is in many sections of the world is used as standard part of the primary healthcare system. Two of the most widely used supplements to combat obesity are not well known in the United States. Rhodiola rosea (Rosavin™) and rhododendron caucasicum, approved for medicinal use in 1969 in Russia by the pharamacological committee of the USSR Ministry of Health, have had over thirty years of clinical study behind them. Rhodiola rosea has been used in Russia and Middle Asia to assist the body in building energy during periods of stress and chronic tension.

Rhodiola rosea assists the function of neurotransmitters, which are what our brain uses to send messages to other cells. Russian scientists have found that, when manipulated, these neurotransmitters have a powerful influence on combating depression, our appetite, our ability to cope with stress, and how well we metabolize (break down) stored fat in adipose (fat) tissue. Rhodiola rosea also known as Golden Root, is a member of the family of plants called crassulaceae, found in the polar arctic regions of Siberia. It is considered as powerful adaptogens, which are substances that greatly enhance your ability to handle various stressors. This phenomenon was first discovered by the renowned Russian physiologist, I.I. Beckman. He gave the classification or critical elements needed by an adaptogen to be able to naturally balance body functions. Siberian ginseng for example is considered to be an adaptogen for its ability to naturally support the body's ability to maintain normal blood-pressure levels.

Dr. Zakir Ramazanov, Ph.D., and Maria de Mar Bernal Suarez, Ph.D., two eminent Russian biochemists, make note of the fact that rhodiola rosea helps eliminate excess or breakdown excess fat already stored in the body while rhododendron caucasicum has the ability to block the absorption of excess fat. Russian scientists have used these preparations to combat obesity and associated problems of excessive body fat with great success. Researchers at the Moscow State Hospital in Russia found that 150mg of rhododendron caucasicum administered three times daily before meals, increased fat excretion up to 15 to 20 percent as compared with a control group.[11]

In addition to the above since 1954, following pharmacological and toxicological clinical trails, the Russian Health Department recommended that specific rhododendron caucasicum plant-based extracts be used to help alleviate chronic venous insufficiency, retinal hemorrhages, circulatory problems and high blood pressure. Dr. Ramazanov and Dr. Suarez state, "both these plant-derived extracts work with natural body mechanisms that stimulate heat (thermogenisis) and speed up the process of diaphoresis."[12] (Diaphoresis is concerned with how effectively your body rids itself of waste, toxins and secretions that enhance the operation of physiological functions.) When using rhodiola rosea according to the Russian Pharmacopea it should be standardized at 0.6 to 1.0% of Rosavin (the most biological active form of its active ingredients).[13]

New Choices in Weight Management

As with all research, there are always further questions to be answered. Although extensive, the preceding review is not exhaustive. There is ongoing worldwide research concerning the efficiency of many other natural alternatives to the existing potentially lethal diet drugs that have emerged. Many of these supplements have been in use for centuries, in varying cultures throughout the world.

Currently, many of these products have moved from an existing auspicious underground entity to acceptable viable options as inclusive remedies in the treatment and prevention of obesity and the maintenance of optimal health here in America. These are truly Nature's biological keys to natural uninhibited mechanisms of weight management and control.

Many products are used extensively throughout the United States and are some of the most popular and best-selling natural fatburners on the market and many are formulated with the natural fatburners discussed in this book. They are listed on the next page for informational purposes only and are not an endorsement by the author. Many can be purchased at local vitamin and drug stores nationwide.

Product Listing:

Aprinol™ (Leptogluterin™)
Anorex ™ (Leptoprin™)
Apple Cider Vinegar
Carb Cutter
Chitosan
Citrimax
Colorade
Dermalin - AP™
Diet Fuel
Dymetadrine
Exercise In A Bottle
Fat Cutter Plus
Fat Trapper
Hydroycut
LipoPeptide
Luprino™ Myoplex
Met Rex or Myoplex Shakes
Metabolife 356
Perfect W-eight™
Stacker 2
Stacker 3
Thermadrene
Thermochrome 3000
(transdermal fat elsifier)
Thermo Genics Plus
Thermo Genics (Quick start)
Thermo Genics
Quick start for men)
The Atkins Shakes, Bars,
Starter Kit
Thyro slim A.M./P.M.
Thyro start

[1] Cichoke, A., "(-) Hydroxycitric Acid: The Revolutionary New Weight Loss Ingredient," Let's Live, July, 1994.

[2] Sullivan, A.C., Triscari, J., "Metabolic Regualtion as a Control for Lipid Disorders. I., Influence of (-) Hydroxycitrate on Experimentally Induced Obesity in the Rodent." Am.J. Clin. Nutr., 30:767-776, 1977.

[3] Lowenstein, J. M., 1971. "Effect of (-) Hydroxycitrate on Fatty Acid Synthesis By Rat Liver in Vivo". J. Biol. Chem. 246:629-632.

[4] Sullivan, A. C., Hamilton, J. G., Miller, O. N., Wheatley, V. R. "Inhibition of Lipogenesis In Rat Liver by (-)Hydroscycitrate," Arch. Biochem. Biophys., 150:183-190, 1972.

[5] Sullivan, A..C. and Triscari, J. "Metabolic Regulation as a Control for Lipid Disorders. I., Influence of (-) Hydroxycitrate on Experimentally Induced Obesity in the Rodent." Am. J. Clin. Nutr., 30:767-776, 1977.

[6] Majeed, M., Citrin: *A Revolutionary Herbal Approach to Weight Management*," New Editions Publishing, Burlingame, CA, 1994, p. 6.

[7] Conte, A., *Clinical Evaluations of (-) Hydroxycitrate Citrin*, New Editions Publishing, Burlingame, CA, 1994.

[8] Ibid, p. 52-60.

[9] Clouatre, D., "Garcinia Cambogia," Whole Foods, October, 1994, p. 56-57.

[10] Conte, A. A., "A Non-prescription Alternative in Weight Reduction Therapy," The Bariatrician, Summer, 1993, p. 17-19

[11] Ramazanov, Z., Suarez, M.M.B., *Effective Natural Stress and Weight Management Using Rhodiola Rosea and Rhododendrom Caucasicum,* ATN/Safe Goods Publishing, Sheffield, MA, 1999.

[12] Ibid.

[13] For more information on these herbs, contact the publisher at (413) 229-7935.

Chapter Eight

Solving the Supplement Puzzle

In the world of supplements, the term "one size fits all", does not apply. Like any well-planned diet and exercise program, you also must choose the right supplement to meet your changing needs. I would strongly suggest that you seek the services of a natural health care professional or someone qualified to give you some insight on the many products available. Additionally, once you have chosen a supplement to enhance your exercise and diet program, keep the following factors in mind:

- **Time:** Give yourself time. These are food supplements and not drugs. In some cases it may take at least thirty days or so to get the nutrient properly circulating in the bloodstream. Dr. Barry Sears in his book *"Enter The Zone"* makes the point concerning consistency and timing. He states that every drug has a therapeutic zone, and for that drug to be effective, you must maintain certain levels of it in the blood stream.[1] The same rule of thumb applies to food supplements.

- **Commitment:** Take your supplements every day. In most cases, it will be necessary to take them with a meal.

- **Follow directions:** As is the case with taking any drug, follow the directions. More is not always better. Stay within the established guidelines, as stipulated on your bottle.

- **Liquid medium:** Do not take your supplements with coffee, tea and/or soda. Take with a full glass of water and/or fruit juice. The notion that heating liquids activates the actions of the ingredients is a misconception.

- **Dependency:** These are natural food supplements and you don't have to worry about becoming addicted. However, you also shouldn't depend on these substances to cover poorly planned diet and exercise regimens. They are designed to augment your efforts, not replace them.

- **Experimentation:** As stated in the opening caption, in the world of supplements, one size doesn't fit all. The great thing about natural supplementation is that it gives you the ability to experiment within limits. It may take you a while to determine which combination or group of products is just right for you. I would, however, recommend that whatever supplements you incorporate into your regimen for weight control, a good multivitamin/ mineral supplement should be considered as your foundation. This should be taken every day with your meals. I would also consider products like lecithin, choline and inositol, fiber, and the lemon and olive oil regimen described in Chapter Six, as standard staples to be included and administered daily.

This author's recommendations:

There are literally thousands of products being researched as possible natural adjuncts to a well balanced diet and exercise program. My extensive list is researched from reports coming in daily citing the benefits of many other compounds.

Acetyl-L-Carnitine
Aloe vera (capsules)
Beta Hydroxy Beta Methylbutyrate (HMB) supplement
Biotin
Borage Oil
Chickweed herb
Conjugated Linoleic Acid supplement
Dandelion herbal capsules or liquid tincture
Evening Primrose Oil
Fennel supplement
Flaxseed Oil
Glucomannan capsules
Griffonia capsules (5-HTP production)
Guarana supplement
Gymnema Sylvestre supplement
Kola Nut herbal supplement
Medium Chain Triglycerides (MCT)
Mustard seeds
Nutritional Yeast
Omega 3 fatty acids
Phosphatidylserine (PS)
Red wine for their polyphenol antioxidants
Uva Ursi supplement
Vanadly Sulfate capsules
Vitamin A, C, E & F (fatty acids)

It is imperative that careful consideration be made in relationship to individual needs, lifestyle and age before incorporating a diet, herb, vitamin or accessory supplement into an existing weight management program. Due to the massive conglomeration of natural diet aids and supplements, this author suggests building a supplement program that focuses on:

- daily needs for long-term usage with requirements for normal maintenance of body systems;
- digestive needs for long-term usage targeting the breakdown of foods for proper assimilation;
- metabolic needs for on-and-off usage to jumpstart sluggish metabolic or fatburning mechanisms;
- energy needs for on-and-off usage for special events or as needed;
- short-term needs (minimal usage to lose a few pounds); and
- fads (the need to experiment) used for the short term as lifestyle changes dictate.

Also, the most important factor concerns percentage of use. Each of these six categories should coincide with the needs of the individual and degree or progress of one's present weight-loss plan. For example, for daily needs, the substances in this section should be stable everyday compounds. This would include:

- multiple vitamin and mineral formulas;
- fiber;
- natural fatburning product or protocol;
- enzymes; and
- amino acids and protein.

The usage here should be a 100 percent dietary inclusion and continued daily for maintenance after you have reached your desired level of weight. The percentage of use in reference to other categories are as follows:

- Daily needs   100%
- Digestive needs   100%
- Metabolic needs   50%
- Mid-term needs   50%
- Short-term needs   15%
- Fad items   5%

It is important that when incorporating supplements into a well- balanced diet and exercise regime, to not just take one vitamin or mineral or a select few. Shari Lieberman, M.A., R.D. author of *Design Your Own Vitamin and Mineral Program* says, "while each has its own biochemical function in the body, nutrients tend to work synergistically (together). In other words, they assist and help their counterparts do their job."[2]

When you put your personal plan together, consider that no two persons require the same substances. Dr. Jeffrey Bland, author of *Assess Your Own Nutritional Status*, maintains that the range of supplement intake required for optimal health may vary from 10 to 100 times from individual to individual. He also expressed the fact that every person possesses some weakness, possibly reducing his or her wellbeing. Dr. Bland suggests, however, going with individual strengths of the patient and working around inherent weakness. The challenge is to understand biochemical individuality, both positive and negative in assessing a proper course of action.[3]

The key factor in administering your supplement intake is to remember "supplements should do just that — supplement the diet, not fill the gaps for poor eating and non-existent exercise and sound nutritional programs," as expressed by Michael Rudolph of the Biology Department of Syracuse University.[4]

---

[1] Sears, B., *Enter The Zone,* Harper and Collins, New York, NY, 1995.

[2] Lieberman, S., Bruning, N., *Design Your Own Vitamin and Mineral Program,* Doubleday and Co., NY, 1980.

[3] Bland, J., *Assess Your Own Nutritional Status,* Keats Publishing, New Canaan, CT., 1987.

[4] Rudolph, M., "Solving the Supplement Puzzle," The Energy Times, Long Beach, CA., 1996

Chapter Nine

Keep Your Backfield In Motion

"Entropy or the second law of Thermodynamics, states that the amount of order in any system left to itself must eventually decrease until complete disorder results. In other words, sit on the sofa long enough, eating junk foods and staring at the TV and you may disintegrate into a puddle of ugly cosmic goo."

Dr. Daniel Mowrey, Ph.D.
"Get Moving," The Energy Times[1]

Recently, the Centers for Disease Control and Prevention recommended that every adult in the United States should accumulate thirty minutes or more of moderate to intensity physical activity on most (and preferably all) days of the week. The new guidelines are intended to complement — not replace — previous advice which has urged at least 20 to 30 minutes or more of vigorous, continuous aerobic exercise three to five times a week. While most of us know that a sound exercise program is vital to maintaining weight, many exercise physiologists contend that Americans do not get enough exercise. Much of what we know about the benefits of exercise is credited to Dr. Kenneth Cooper, known as the father of exercise. Dr. Cooper, founder and director of the prestigious Cooper Wellness Center in Dallas, Texas is cited as the person most responsible for getting America moving — running that is. Dr. Cooper has written four landmark books, *Aerobics, The New Aerobics, Aerobics for Women* and *The Aerobic Way.* According to Charles T. Kurtzleman, former National Director of the Fitness Finders Program and the Editor of Consumer Guide, "Kenneth Cooper has done more to popularize cardiovascular exercise that any other person in the world."

Today, because of the efforts of pioneers like Dr. Cooper, we now know that lack of exercise contributes to many negative degenerative complications such as heart disease, chronic fatigue, stroke, Type II diabetes, colon cancer, osteoporosis, osteoarthritis pain and inflammation, hypercholesterolemia (elevated LDL cholesterol levels) and obesity. Although the health benefits of regular exercise are enormous, it is advisable to check with your personal physician before starting any exercise program. Physical exertion can trigger the onset of acute myocardial infarction (heart attack), especially in persons who maintain sedentary lifestyles. The risk of infarction is considerably less among people who have reported participating in regular exercise at least five times per week with periods of heavy physical exertion six times per week.

Concerning most cases of obesity, the real problem begins with the amount of calories used when not exercising. Muscle cells are fairly active and are busy all the time. On the other hand, fat cells are fairly inactive and don't contain nearly as many blood vessels as a result of failing to maintain physical activity. Because of this, many fitness and health experts conclude that a portion of your activity level should be geared toward building muscle. Pound for pound, muscle keeps your metabolic rate on high, even while you sleep. Your metabolic rate determines how fast or well your body is utilizing the calories you take in.

It is imperative that you get approval from your personal physician before starting any exercise program. He or she will probably have you undergo a complete physical examination and a stress test (EKG) to determine the strength of your heart at various levels of physical exertion. Once your health professional has given you the go-ahead, you will have to choose what type of exercise is best suited for you. No matter which activity you choose, you need to keep one thing in mind — **start out slow!** Moving too quickly into your new routine can cause injuries to muscles that are not used to being manipulated. Exercise physiologists recommend that you begin with 10 to 15 minutes of moderate activity per day, gradually increasing the time and intensity of the endeavor.

Choosing the right exercise is of vital importance. As we age, subtle internal changes occur on an ongoing basis.

- Your heart's ability to pump blood has decreased one percent per year since age thirty.
- Your blood vessels tend to narrow as you age and as such blood flow from the arms to the legs is as much as 60 percent slower at age 60 than 25.
- The levels of your muscle power diminish as much as 30 percent at age 60 from its levels recorded at age 25.
- Furthermore, as we age the walls of our chest can stiffen, causing the maximum amount of oxygen we are able to use to decrease by 29 percent in men and up to 50 percent in women.[2]

It is important to remember that without proper exercise, diet and a commitment to the future, you will never reach or sustain permanent weight/fat loss goals. Your program should work well apart from diet pills, natural fatburners, and the loss of poundage. A total fitness program may initiate a positive change in the following areas:

- Aerobic (using oxygen) capacity of your lungs and heart muscle
- Flexibility of your muscles
- Muscle building process
- Strength of your bone and muscle structure

Whatever your exercise activity of choice is, be consistent and make it fun. For your exercise program to be effective, especially for weight loss, your routine or workout has to go to the point where fat begins to be burned. This occurs when metabolism (the rate at which your body uses or burns up calories) switches to fat-burning after about forty minutes of exercise. Losing one pound of fat means metabolizing about 3,500 calories. Running one mile burns about 100 calories. According to Dr. Earl Mindell it is better to concentrate on long, slow deliberate and repetitive activities. He maintains that it is the long slow distance work that turns on the fat-burning processes.[3] Research has shown that this type of exercise can stimulate continual fatburning several hours after the session is over. It may be advisable to sit down and re-think when and how often some of your most enjoyable activities occur and turn them into calorie-burning sessions. The Surgeon General now recommends that every American start expending 150 calories a day through such activities as gardening, leisurely strolls, cycling, walking your dog and other physical activities.

The following chart will give you an idea of how you can potentially burn up to 150 calories in 15 to 45 minutes of physical activity:

DAILY ACTIVITY	TIME (minutes)
Washing/waxing car	45-60
Washing windows/floors	45-60
Volleyball	45
Touch football	30-45
Gardening	30-45
Wheeling a wheelchair	20-40
Basketball (shooting baskets)	35
Bicycling 5 miles	30
Dancing (fast)	30
Pushing a stroller 1.5 miles	30
Raking leaves	30
Walking 2 miles	30
Water aerobics	30
Swimming laps	20
Wheelchair basketball	20
Basketball (playing game)	15-20
Jumping rope	15
Running	15
Shoveling snow	15
Stair walking	15

Figure 6.1: Calories Used in 15-45 minutes of Various Activities. Adapted from Surgeon General's report on Physical Activity and Health as found on the web at the following address: (www.cdegov/nccdphp/sgr/htm)

To reap the long-term benefit of an overall fitness program, Dr. Stuart Berger, author of *Forever Young*, maintains that you should focus your physical lifestyle changes not merely on the weight loss, but on longevity. He insists that you should become an activist, not an athlete, and that regular activity, not just strenuous exercise, is the key to weight management, health and longevity.[4] In fact, based on epidemiological studies done in relationship to the degree of activity or exercise level, the greatest benefit comes when you change from no activity to moderate activity rather than from moderate activity to high activity. A total well-being program can give you the following benefits: more personal energy, more enjoyable and active leisure time, greater ability to handle domestic and job-related stress, less depression, less hypochondria (imaginary ill-health) and less free-floating anxiety, fewer physical complaints, more efficient digestion, less constipation, a better self-image, more self-confidence, a more attractive, streamlined body and more effective personal weight control, easier pregnancy and childbirth and a slowing of the aging process.[5]

> *Exercise and moderation perpetuate and maintain something of our early vigor even in old age.*
> Cicero, 44 B.C.[6]

Although the list on the previous page contains only a few of the benefits of a total fitness program, the long-term rewards have far-reaching implications. The key to any sound program is consistency. Individuals who maintain established weight guidelines usually have an action plan in place. To keep focused on your intended goals and move yourself away from negative lifestyle tendencies, you can try the following:
• forget the notion that skills are a prerequisite for fitness;
• become involved with a club or class;
• start at your own level;
• be prepared for subtle changes at first;
• revel in the psychological benefits, not just the physical;
• celebrate milestones big and small with meaningful rewards;
• set goals within your reach;
• find a nag or partner;
• lean on friends and family for help;
• add more of what inspires you (music, etc.); and
• turn daily chores and activities into workouts.[7]

Ninety-five percent of Americans regain their lost weight, often within a year.[8] People's individual mindset differentiates those who successfully manage their weight from those who habitually relapse into unhealthy dietary and sedentary lifestyles. Additionally, Cathy Nonas, M.S.R.D., Director of the Vantallie Center for Nutrition and Weight Management at St. Luke's Roosevelt Hospital in New York City contends that individuals who gain a few pounds realize that this is a part of weight maintenance. She believes that this occurrence should be viewed as an opportunity to re-establish your priorities and your present weight maintenance plan. My recommendation to help yourself achieve long-term weight and fat loss goals, as well as maintain a state of perpetual health to boot, is to keep your backfield in motion!

[1] Mowrey, D., "Get Moving," The Energy Times, Long Beach, CA., 1:96:50-56.

[2] Berger, S.M., *Forever Young*, William Morrow and Co., New York, NY, 1989.

[3] Mindell, E., *What You Should Know About Better Nutrition For Athletes*, Keats Publishing, New Canaan CT, 1996.

[4] Berger, S.M., *Forever Young*, William Morrow and Co.,NY, 1989.

[5] Cooper, K1H., The Aerobics Program For Total Well-Being, Bantam Books, NY, 1982.

[6] Renau, K., "Making The Case For Exercise," Healthwatch, Louisville, KY, July/Aug. 1991, p. 64-65.

[7] Mc Mahon, B., "There's No Stopping You," The Walking Magazine, Boston MA, May, 1997.

[8] Stephen Guillo, Ph.D.,*Thin Taste Better,* Carol Southern Books, 1995.

Chapter Ten

Managing Your Fat Burning

You must be willing to commit yourself to a lifelong weight control program. Don't be alarmed by the sound of a lifelong program. Almost everyone practices some form of weight control throughout life. To maintain a desired weight instead of going up or down, you will simply be more aware of your program, at least initially. Even as you begin to work toward your desired weight, it is important to set up a nutritionally balanced diet and activity plan that you feel good about and can make a routine part of your life.

Dr. Jack D. Osman
Associate Professor of Health Science
Towson State University, Baltimore MD

When you review the comments above by Dr. Osman, they imply your plan should ensures that your general lifestyle is well balanced, both nutritionally and physically, and one that is both enjoyable and mentally satisfying. I am suggesting that you follow what obesity researchers term the 25-50-25 rule. By making this rule part of your lifelong dietary habits you will have a better chance of controlling your weight and fatburning capabilities.

The 25-50-25 PLAN calls for you to consume:
- 25 percent of your daily calories at breakfast
- 50 percent at lunchtime
- the final 25 percent at dinnertime

According to Dr. Lawrence E. Lamb, M.D., former Professor of Medicine at Baylor University and Chief of Medical Science at the School of Aerospace Medicine states that, "the problem with most obesity treatment programs is that they are not designed to treat the real cause." Dr. Lamb maintains that we often engage ourselves with "symptomatic treatment."[1] For example, if a person is fat, the weight loss plan to attack the symptom is composed of reducing the amount of food intake or resorting to dangerous diet drugs. While this approach is commonly accepted, used and self-administered in many cases, it may not be addressing the underlying cause. In this case, once this symptomatic treatment is stopped, weight gain reoccurs. The real problem has not been addressed. As cited by Dr. Lamb most people get fat while continuing to eat about the same thing they ate in earlier years and while doing about the same amount of physical activity. The real problem with obesity in many cases (beyond genetics) lies in how many calories you are using while doing nothing, not while you are exercising.[2]

A Simple Plan

Lifelong sounds imposing, but the key to managing your weight and fat loss goals is in what you do today, this minute, this hour. Focus on today, keep it simple and give yourself time. Don't focus on where you are but where you are headed. By devising a simple plan of action, you will be well on your way to reaching — but more importantly maintaining — your weight loss goals for life. You may want to follow the guidelines below that are very easy to self manage and alter them as needed.

A Small Master plan
- Utilize the 25-50-25 rule of eating.
- Keep your backfield in motion.
- Utilize and interchange the natural protocols, accessory and fat-burning supplements.
- Avoid fad diets.

Additional steps you may take to assist you in your efforts follow. Utilize as many of the suggestions as you can. Please remember these suggestions are not written in stone. Interchange and utilize the combinations that are right for you.

75 Ways to Reduce Weight Safely and Naturally
1. Stay active – Keep moving;
2. Watch your fat intake;
3. Follow the 25-50-25 rule;
4. Alter your exercise;
5. Drink 8 to 10 glasses of ice-cold water daily;
6. Know you correct calorie ratio;
7. Reduce stress and do not eat during stressful episodes;
8. Don't consume large meals after 8 P.M.;

9. Don't restrict calories, eat in moderation and do not skip meals;
10. Concentrate on overall health;
11. Eat smaller meals;
12. Eliminate unhealthy lifestyle choices;
13. Consider fasting periodically;
14. Consume at least 25 grams of fiber a day;
15. Reduce the amount of time you watch TV;
16. Incorporate the use of natural fatburners into your weight and fat loss program;
17. Seek professional help;
18. Increase your vegetable intake;
19. Consume more complex carbohydrates;
20. Avoid sugary snacks and foods;
21. Use only lean cuts of meat;
22. Remove sugar, and white flour from your diet;
23. Reduce your salt intake;
24. Have regular checkups (have your thyroid gland activity checked too);
25. Stay away from hydrogenated oils;
26. Love thyself;
27. Have sex regularly;
28. Join a fitness club;
29. Avoid simple carbohydrates;
30. Make protein your last snack of the day;
31. Keep your colon cleansed;
32. Utilize cleansing herbs in your supplement program;
33. Walk daily; you don't necessarily have to run;
34. Evaluate your plan of action and make changes as necessary;
35. Give yourself time. If you lose a pound a week you will be 52 pounds lighter by year's end;
36. Be realistic in setting your weight- and fat-loss goals;
37. Do not use food to alleviate stress, use the energy having sex or for working out;
38. Find a buddy and become a weight-loss team;
39. Get plenty of sleep;
40. Resist the temptation for quick fixes;
41. Learn as much as you can about the Glycemic Index of Foods;
42. Eat to supply fuel for an anticipated activity not for what you just did;
43. Do not totally cut out fat in your diet — you need some fat to initiate lipolysis (the breakdown of fat);

44. Take a multiple enzyme formula daily;
45. Consume one to two tablespoons of medium chain triglycerides daily;
46. Keep carbohydrates intake at 300 to 400 grams daily;
47. Be persistent. Expect subtle changes, not extreme ones;
48. Start out with a fitness plan or activity you like or have some level of skill in;
49. Learn new hobbies;
50. Drink alcoholic beverages in moderation;
51. Eliminate fried food;
52. Identify your key weight loss problem: appetite control, metabolism, snacking, blood sugar abnormalities, and take action to correct it;
53. Consider attributes of weight training;
54. Seek out friends and family members who have similar interest and goals;
55. Stay away from fad diets;
56. Get plenty of rest;
57. Consider attributes of natural hormones;
58. Toss self-defeating habits and attitude out the window;
59. Be committed in your efforts;
60. If you get off track start over the next day;
61. Accept criticism be honest with your efforts;
62. Monitor daily eating habits focus on today;
63. Change shopping habits, shop on a full stomach and don't buy fattening snacks;
64. Go ahead treat yourself today — you've earned it;
65. Monitor your portions. Don't overload your plate;
66. Drink a full 8oz glass of water before meals;
67. Practice exchanging healthy foods for less desirable ones;
68. Stop eating once you're full;
69. Check your weight periodically. Monitor your progress;
70. Don't be too rigid with your weight and your fat loss plans — flexibility is the key;
71. Eat a variety of foods;
72. Accept who you are work toward your goals;
73. Be patient;
74. Learn a new skill;
75. Use olive oil and a lemon cleanse to keep your liver free of fatty deposits.

In the next chapter, you will find listings of web sites, health and fitness clubs as well as various weight loss centers and organizations that can help you.

You Are In Control

It is important that you understand that the most important piece of this puzzle is you. Maintaining the sleek slender look you desire can be achieved safely and effectively without the use of dangerous diet drugs. The key, however, is not in just balancing your diet; it requires a lifelong balance of self-direction. This you control.

A new challenge is facing those within the healthcare arena and the American people, and that challenge is to resist becoming mere reflections of the technology that surrounds us. The call for quick temporary fixes may in the long run be less beneficial for the patient and an unhealthy option. Resist the notion that optimal health can be equated with "not hurting," and resist the continued trend of practicing treatment versus prevention. It is within these parameters that we as health care professionals must find a way to bridge the gap as expressed by Dr. Anthony Conte, M.D., a renowned Bariatrie (Obesity) Physician and researcher.

> *While some state medical boards allow physicians to prescribe appetite depressants for a maximum of twelve weeks out of the year, regardless of successful management and benefits to the obese patient, I am a firm believer in the new age of alternative medicine which is rapidly catching on. Physicians need effective and safe medications for obesity. Pharmaceutical firms, scientists and health care professional, must recognize that herbal medicine should be considered an equal partner and not an adversary.* [3]

Good Luck and, As Always, Good Health To You!

---

[1] Lamb, L.E., Metobolics: Putting Your Food Energy To Work, Harper and Row, NY, 1974.

[2] Ibid, p.245-258

[3] Passwater, R.A. "America's No. 1 Health Problem – Overweight but Undernourished: An Interview with Dr. Anthony Conte," Whole Foods Magazine, Plainfield, NJ, Oct 1996, p. 48-57.

Chapter Eleven

Holistic Health, Weight-and Fat-Loss Directory

In this section, you will find a number of web sites, weight loss and fitness centers, as well as various organizations all designed to help you achieve your weight-and fat-loss goals.

Organizations

American Association of Lifestyle Counselors
P.O. Box 610412
Dept. 55
Dallas, TX 75261-0410
(817) 545-3220

National Institute of Diabetes and
Digestive and Kidney Diseases (NIDDK)
National Institute of Health
31 Center Drive
MSC 2560
Bethesda, MD 20892-2560
http://www.niddk.nih.gov/health/nutri/nutrit.html

Overeaters Anonymous Inc.
World Service Office
6075 Zenith Court NE
Rio Ranch, NM 87124
(505) 891-4320
http://www.overeatersanonymous.org

Weight Watchers International
(800) 651-6000
http://www.weightwatchers.com
The Institute of Health Solutions
1623 A Fifth Ave.
San Rafael, CA 94901
(415) 457-3369 (Live Support)
http://www.weightsolution.com

Web Sites

Bodyweightloss.com-natural weight loss
http://www.bodyweightloss.com/about.htlml

Diet Center Worldwide, Inc.
http://www.dietcenter.com

Dietinfo.com
http://www.dietinfo.com

Dr. Atkins, The Atkins Diet
http://www.atkinscenter.com

Duke University Diet and Fitness
http://www.mc.duke.edu.dfc.home.html

Ephedra Herbal Information Center
http://www.kcweb.com/herblephedra.html

Fitness Connection – Weight Loss:
Clinics and Consultants
http://fitconnection.com/directory/weight-
loss/clinics_and_consultants/index.shtml

Herbal Life
http://www.marketingservice.net/daretobethin/recipes.html

Klein-Becker USA
Free personalized weight loss plan
http://www.myfreediet.com

Learn Education Center
http://www.learneducation.com

Nutrisystem.com
http://nutrisystem.com

US City Network Directory:
Weight Management: Products
http://alaska.uscity.net/weight_managment/products

Weight Loss Programs
http://www.dietquik.com/p101html

Weight Loss Centers

Coastal Medical Weight Loss Centers
7061 Clainemont Mesa Blvd.
Suite 202
San Diego, CA 92111
(800) 884-slim or (858) 277-6751
http://www.coastmed.signonsandiego.com/

LA Weight Loss Centers
2091 Blackhorse Pike
Turnersville, NJ 08012
(800) 331-4035 or (856) 728- 4341
http://www.laweightloss.com/

Jenny Craig International
11355 N. Torrey Pines Road
LaJolla, CA 92038
(800) 597-Jenny or (858) 812-7000
http://www.jennycraig.com/

Physcians Weight Loss Centers
395 Springside Drive
Akron, OH
(800) 440-7952 or (330) 666-7952
http://www.pwlc.com/

Test America Medical Weight Loss Center
3603 State Street
Santa Barbara, CA 93105
(805) 563-3301
http://www.testamerica.com

Last Words

An Open Letter To Healthcare Professionals

Restoring Our Sense of Direction

In the coming years, a new model must be established which fosters clear and concise guidelines that will move the American public toward sound nutritional practice versus gadgets, fads and total chemical dependence. Emerging natural weight management programs should not only consider weight-and fat-loss management they should also focus on neurotransmitter — receptor interaction. These receptor sites directly influence mood, appetite, metabolism, energy, and other functions related to weight management. There is an exquisite balance between the brain and the nervous system. It is a network of chemical keys, signals and switches that modulate this unique communication system. Conversely, what each individual eats and drinks may affect the production and action of these brain neurotransmitters.

A major shift needs to manifest itself that also will move individuals toward developing short-term interchangeable goals, that will initiate long-term natural habitual tendencies with a strong emphasis on self reliance, versus diet drug usage and dependence. Finally, all actions toward weight management should focus on life extension, due to the fact that data conclusively shows that:

The very obese die earlier than the very slender.
-Hippocrates

Diet Drug Warning

WYETH-AYERST ®**W** *LABORATORIES*

P.O. BOX 8299, PHILADELPHIA, PA 19101-8299   *Division of American Home Products Corporation*

Philip J. de Vane, M.D.
Vice President, Clinical Affairs
and North American Medical Director

> Re: Plegine® (phendimetrazine tartrate tablets)
> WARNING regarding Valvular Irregularities and Primary Pulmonary Hypertension

Dear Health Care Professional:

Wyeth-Ayerst Laboratories, Division of American Home Products Corporation, wants to call your attention to a new warning added to the labeling of Plegine® (phendimetrazine tartrate tablets) The boxed warning states:

Anorexigens have been reported to be associated with the occurrence of serious regurgitant cardiac valvular disease, including disease of the mitral, aortic, and/or tricuspid valves. In one literature report, 24 patients, who received combination therapy with fenfluramine and phentermine for treatment of obesity, were found to have regurgitant cardiac valvular disease; five of these patients required valvular surgery. The valves of these five patients were found to have a gross pathologic and/or histologic appearance resembling that seen in patients with alterations in serotonin metabolism. In these reports and other reported cases, fenfluramine was taken generally in combination with phentermine. However, there are some reports in which valvular disease was seen in patients taking fenfluramine alone.

Primary pulmonary hypertension (PPH) – a rare, frequently fatal disease of the lungs – has been found to occur with increased frequency in patients receiving anorexigens. **(See WARNINGS.)**

There have been reports of PPH and valvular irregularities in users of Plegine (phendimetrazine tartrate tablets).

The safety and effectiveness of the combined use of Plegine with other anorexigens in the treatment of obesity have not been established, and there is no approved use of these products together in the treatment of obesity. Plegine is approved only as a single agent for short-term use (i.e., a few weeks).

Wyeth-Ayerst has received information concerning patients who had taken phendimetrazine and experienced valvular abnormalities and/or primary pulmonary hypertension. It appears that all patients had a history of using at least one other anorexigen. Since the removal of Pondimin® (fenfluramine hydrochloride tablets) C-IV and Redux™ (dexfenfluramine hydrochloride capsules) C-IV from the market in September 1997, there have been reports that physicians are prescribing phendimetrazine in combination with phentermine in a limited number of cases. We emphasize that such concomitant use is not indicated.

In light of this information, Wyeth-Ayerst would like to remind you of two important points in connection with phendimetrazine products, including Plegine℗ (phendimetrazine tartrate tablets):

• Phendimetrazine is not indicated for concomitant use with any other anorexigenic drug. Wyeth-Ayerst does not recommend such concomitant use and does not know of any adequate and well-controlled studies demonstrating the safety and effectiveness of these drugs when used in combination.

• Phendimetrazine is not indicated for long-term use. The labeling clearly states that it is indicated only for short-term use of a few weeks.

Sincerely,

Philip J. de Vane, M.D.

INDEX

Bibliography

-Adams, R., Murray, F., *All You Should Know About Health Foods*, Larchmont Books, NY, 1975.

-Airola, Paavo, N. D., Ph.D., *The Miracle of Garlic*, Phoenix AZ: Health Plus Publishers, 1986.

-Airola, Paavo, N. D., Ph.D., *Are You Confused*, Health Plus Publishers, Phoenix, AZ, 1971.

-Anderson, J.W., Johnstone, B.M., Cook-Newell, M.E., "Meta-analysis of effects of soy protein intake on serum lipids in humans," New England Journal of Medicine, 1995, 333:276-282.

-Aoyama, T. et.al., "Soy protein isolate and its hydrolysate reduce body fat of dietary obese rats and genetically obese mice," Nutrition 2000, May: 16 (5): 349.

-Apovian, C.M., "The Use of Pharmacologic Agents In the Treatment of The Obese Patient," The Journal of The American Osteopathic Association, Vol. 99, No. 10 Part 2, October 1999, p.52-55.

-Atkins, R.C., *Dr. Atkins New Diet Revolution*, Avon Books, New York, NY 1999.

-Barnard, N., *Foods That Cause You To Lose Weight*, The Magni Group, McKinney, TX, 1992.

-Bettger, W. J., O'Dell, B. L., "A Critical Physiological Role of Zinc In The Structure and Function of Bio-Membranes," Life Sciences, 1981; 28:1425-1438.

-Bland, J., *Assess Your Own Nutritional Status*, Keats Publishing, New Canaan, CT, 1987.

-Bland, J., *Digestive Enzymes*, Keats Publishing, New Canaan, CT, 1993.

-Bland, J., *Octacosanol, Carnitine and Other Accessory Nutrients*, Keats Publishing, New Canaan, CT, 1982.

-Bliznakov, E.G., Hunt, G.L., *The Miracle Nutrient Coenzyme CoQ10*, Bantam Books, NY, 1986.

-Block W., et al., "Depression, Anxiety and Sleep Breakthrough," Life Enhancement, Petaluma, CA, Issue No. 27, 11:96: p. 2.

-Blum, I, Vered, Y., Graff, E., et.al, "The influence of meal composition on plasma serotonin and norepinephrine concentration." Metabolism, 1992: 41 (2): 137-140.

-Brainum, J., Melatonin "The Better To Sleep With", Muscle and Fitness, Woodland Hills, CA, 3:95: 218-220.

Brown, D. J., "Aging Healthfully, Herbs For Health," Interweave Press, Loveland, CO, September 10, 1997, p. 40-45.

-Burroughs, A., *The Master Cleaner*, Burroughs Books, Auburn, CA, 1993.

-Butterworth, C. E., "Ascorbate - Cholesterol - Letchin Interactions: Factors of Potential Importance In Pathogenesis of Atheroselerosis," American Journal of Clinical Nutrition, 8; 74:866-76.

-Campbell, R. A., *Biology 3rd Edition*, Benjamin Cummings, Redwood City, CA, 1993.

-Carper, J. *The Food Pharmacy*, Bantam Books, NY, 1988.

-Challem, L. L., *Spirulina*, Keats Publishing, New Canaan, CT, 1981, p. 2.

-Chang, M. L. W., and Johnson, M.A., "Effect of Garlic on Carbohydrate Metabolism and Lipid Syntheses in Rats," Journal of Nutrition, 110:931, 1980.

-Cichoke, A., "(-) Hydroxycitric Acid: The Revolutionary New Weight Loss Ingredient," Let's Live, July 1994.

-Citrimax Makes News, Health Foods Business, October 1994, p. 5.

-Clive, T., "Brave New Drug World, Can Phen-Fen Really Make You Thinner?" Iron Man Magazine, Oxnard Ca., Feb., 1997, p.102-103.

-Clouatre, D., *Anti-Fat Nutrients,* Pax Publishing, San Francisco, CA, 1997.

-Clouatre, D., Garcinia Cambogia, Whole Foods, October 1994, p. 56-57.

-"Coenzyme Q10" American Institute for Biosocial Research, Life Sciences Division - Botanical Medical Series No. 4, Tacoma, WA, 1987.

-Conte, A. A., "A Non-prescription Alternative in Weight Reduction Therapy," The Bariatrician, Summer 1993, p. 17-19.

-Conte, A., *Clinical Evaluations of (-) Hydroxycitrate Citrin,* New Editions Publishings, Burlingame, CA, 1994.

-"CoQ10 and Cardiovascular Disease," The Energy Times Medicine Chest Long Beach, CA, Jan./Feb., 1995, pg. 55-56.

-Cowley, G., "Melatonin," Newsweek, New York, NY, 10:95: 46-49.

-Crosby, S.W., "How To Thrive On An Ailing Planet," Ms Fitness Magazine, Corona CA, Summer 1997, p.76-78.

-Curtis, H., *Biology,* Worth Publishing, New York, NY, 1983.

-Deuch, K., Kanauchi, O., Shizukurshi, M., Kobayahsi, E., "Continuous and Massive Intake of Chitosan Affects Mineral and Fat-Soluble, Vitamin Status in Rats Fed On A High Fat Diet", Bioscience, Biochem, July 1995, 59(7): 1211-6.

-Despre S., et.al., "Level of Physical Fitness and Adipocyte Lipolysis in Humans," Applied Physiology, Respiratory, Environmental and Exercise Physiology, (56) 1984,: 1157-1161.

-Drake, D., Uhlman, M., *Making Medicine Making Money,* Andrew and McMeel Publishing, NY, 1993.

-Duchane, D., "Lower Body Fat: You Know About Beta Agonists," Muscle Media, 2000, Golden, CO, 10:963, 94-99.

-Dunne, L. J., *Nutrition Almanac,* 4th Ed., McGraw Hill, NY, 1990, p. 74.

-Eckstein, E. F., *Food, People and Nutrition,* Avi Publishing, Westport, CT, 1980.

-Edelstein, B., *The Underburner's Diet: How To Rid Your Body of Excess -Fat Forever,* MacMillan Publishing, NY, 1987

-"Ephedrine Products Become OTC in Nebraska," Health Supplement Retailer, Virgo Publishing, Phoenix Az., Vol. 7. No. 6, June, 2001, p.7.

-Evans, G. W., *The Picolinates, How They Help Build Muscle Without Steriods,* Keats Publishing, New Canaan, CT, 1989.

-Fahey, T. D., "DHEA," Muscle and Fitness, Woodland Hills, CA., 1995: 8:94-97.

-Fahey, T.D., "Obesity In America" Body Mass Index and Obesity, Muscular Development" Vol. 37, No. 2 Feb., 2000, p.62-63.

-Farago, P., Lagnado, J., *Life in Action,* Alfred A. Knopf, NY, 1972, pg. 99.

-Farguar, J.W., *The American Way of Life Need Not Be Hazardous To Your Health,* Stanford Alumni Assoc., Stanford CA, 1987.

-Fellman, B., A. "Clockwork Gland," Science, 856 (4): 76-81.

-Ferguson, J.M., *Habits Not Diets,* Bull Publishing Co., Palo Alto CA, 1988.

-Fernstrom, J., "Acute and chronic effects of protein and carbohydrate injection on brain tryptophan levels and serotonin sysnthesis," Nutrition Review, May 1986, 44: 25-36.

-Fisher, J.A., *The Chromium Program,* Harper and Row, NY, 1990.

-Folkers, K., et al., "Biomedical and Clinical Aspects of Coenzyme Q" (Vol. 1) Eisenvier Science Publishers 1977, 1980, 1981, 1984.

-Foster, S., "Garcinia Cambogia" Health Foods Business, June 1994, p. 27.

-Foster, S., "The Misunderstood Herb," Herbs For Health, Vol. 9 No. 2, Loveland CO, Dec. 1996/Jan. 1997.

-Foster, S., "Top Notch Herbs and Immunostimulants," Better Nutrition, Atlanta, GA, 10:95:60-67.

-Fox, M., Stanten, M., "Diet Pills Boom or Bust?" Prevention Magazine, Emmas PA, April 1997, Vol. 49, No. 4, p. 92-95.

-Fredericks, C., Carlton Fredericks, *Nutrition Guide for the Prevention and Cure of Common Ailments and Diseases*, Simon and Schuster, NY, 1982.

-"Garlic Ancient Wisdom for Today's Healing," Better Nutrition, Atlanta, GA, 10:95:16.

-Garattini, S., Bizzi, A., Caccia, C., et.al., "Progress in assessing the role of serotonin in the control of food intake," Clinical Neuropharmacology, 1988: 11 (Suppl): S8-S32.

-Garrison, R., Somer, E., *The Nutrition Desk Reference*, Keats Publishing, New Canaan, CT, 1995.

-Gibbs, et al., "Phenylalanine," Reviews in Clinical Nutrition, 1982, Vol. 2., p. 53-59.

Goodhart, R., Shils, M., *Modern Nutrition In Health and Disease*, Lea and Febiger, Philadelphia, PA, 1980.

-Gottlieb, B., *New Choices In Natural Healing*, Rodale Press, Emmaus, PA, 1995.

-Guyton, A. C., *Function of the Human Body*, W. B., Saunders, Philadelphia, PA, 1969, p. 397.

-Haas, R., *Eat Smart, Think Smart*, Harper Collins, NY, 1993.

-Haas, R., "Redux and Fen-phen: Deadly Diet Drugs Removed From the Market," All Muscular Development, Ronkonkoma, NY, March 1998, p. 188-189.

-Haas, R., "Yo Yo Dieting Linked To Cancer," All Natural Muscular Development, Ronkokoman, NY, Sept. 1997, p. 168.

-Haussinger, D. et.al., "The Role Of Cellular Hydration in The Regulation of Cell Function," Journal of Biochemistry, 313 (1996): 697-710.

-Health Watch, "Hot Diet Pills Are Prescription For Complications and Disappointment," Let's Live Magazine, Los Angeles, Ca. April 1997, p. 23.

-Hendler, S. S., *The Complete Guide To Anti-Aging Nutrients*, Simon and Schuster, NY, 1985, p. 191.

-Hunger P., "Basic Mechanisms and Clinical Implications," *Raven Press*, NY, p. 115-125, 1976.

-"Industry Berates U.S. News Supplement Coverage," Health Supplement Retailer, Virgo Publishing, Phoenix, AZ., Vol. 7 No. 6 June, 2001, p.7.

-Jensen, B.C., *Tissue Cleansing Through Bowel Management*, Bernard Jensen Publications, Esconidido CA, 1981.

-Jordon, P., "Neuroendocrinology" American Fitness Magazine, Sherman Oaks, Ca., May/June 1988. p.38-40.

-Katahn, M., *Beyond Diet, The 28-Day Metobolic Breakthrough Plan*, Berkley Books, NY, 1984.

-Katahn, M., *One Meal at A Time*, W.W. Norton and Co., NY, 1991.

-Katahn, M., *The Rotation Diet*, Bantam Books,NY, 1986.

-Kawano-Takahashi Y., et.al., "Effect of Soy A Saponing On Gold Thioglucose (GTG) Induced Obesity in Mice, Internal Journal of Obesity 1986; 10(4): 293-302.

-Keane, M., *The Red Yeast Rice Cholesterol Solution,* Adams Media Corporation, Holbrook, MA, 1999.

-King, S.J., "Retailers Gain Sales With Natural Weight Loss Aids," Whole Foods Magazine, Plainfield NJ Vol. 17, No. 3 March 1994, p. 37-46.

-Kloss, J., *Back To Eden,* Back To Eden Publishing, Loma Linda, CA, 1988.

-Knox, A. "Relying On Pills To Pull The Weight, Phila. Inquirer, Phila. PA, 1997.

-Kramer, P. D., *Listening to Prozac,* Viking Press, NY, 1993.

-Kritchevsky, D., et al., "Influence of Garlic Oil on Cholesterol Metabolism in Rats." Nutrition Reports International, 22:641-645, 1980.

-Kuntzleman, C.T., *Rating The Exercises,* William Morrow and Co., NY, 1978.

-Lamb, L.E., *Metabolics: Putting Your Food Energy To Work,* Harper and Row, NY, 1974.

-Lavau and Hashim, "Effect of Medium Chain Triglyceride on Lipogenesis and Body Fat in The Rat," Journal of Nutrition, (108), 1978: 613-620.

-Le Monick, M.D., "The New Miracle Drug," Time Magazine, Sept. 23, 1996, p.61-67.

-Levine, H., "Fen-phen Killed My Wife," Cosmopolitan Magazine, December 1997, p.196-199.

-Lewis Laboratories International, Letchin: "A Powerful Nutritional Factor-Vital to Both Mind and Body," Natural Remedies, Stamford, CT, March, 1997, p.5-7.

-Lowenstein, J. M., 1971. "Effect of (-) Hydroxycitrate on Fatty Acid Synthesis by Rat Liver in Vivo," J. Biol Chem, 246:629-632.

-Majeed, M., Citrin, *A Revolutionary Herbal Approach to Weight Management,* New Editions Publishing, Burlingame, CA, 1994.

-Marley, W.P., *Health and Fitness,* Saunders College Publishing, Phila. PA, 1982.

-Martin, D. W., Mayers, P. A., Rodwell, V. W., *Harper's Review of Biochemistry,* 19th Edition, pg. 51-52 Lange Medical Publications, Los Altos CA, 1983.

-Mathura, C. B., Singh, H. H., Tizabi, Y., Hughes, J. E., Flesher, S. A., "Effects of Chronic Tryptophan Loading on Serotonin (5ht) Levels In Neonatal Rat Brain," Journal of American Medical Association, 1986; 78 (7): 645.

-Mason, J.E., Faich, G.A. "Pharmacotheraphy For Obesity-Do The Benefits Out-weight the Risk?" New England Journal of Medicine, 8:29:1996, 335 (9) 659-60.

-Mayer, J., *Human Nutrition,* Springfield, IL, Charles C. Thomas, 1974.

-McAfee, L., Redux: "Is Weight Loss Worth It?" *Labyrinth, The Philadelphia Women's Newspaper,* Westbury Publishing Inc., Phila. PA: Vol. 15, No 1 1997.

-McArdle, W.D., Mage, J.R., *Weight Management Diet and Exercise, Found in Medical Applications of Clinical Nutrition,* Edited by Jeffrey Bland, Keats Publishing, New Canaan CT, 1983, p.99-132.

-McClain, C., et al., "Zinc Status Before and After Zinc Supplementation Of Eating Disorder Patients," Journal of American College of Nutrition, 1992; 11:694.

-McNutt, K. W., McNutt, D. R., *Nutrition and Food Choices,* Science Research Associated, 1978. p. 84.

-Mc Phee, S.J., Schroeder, S.A., *Current Medical Diagnosis and Treatment,* Appleton and Lange, Stanford, CA, 1996.

-Mercer, E. H., *Cells: Their Structure and Function,* Doubleday and Co., NY, 1962.

-The Merck Manual, 14th Ed., Merck, Sharp and Dohme Research Laboratories, Rahway NJ, 1982, pp. 997-1012.

-Miller, B., *Fiber The Vital Missing Link,* Bruce Miller Enterprises, Inc., Dallas, TX, 1992.

-Miller, D.S., Parsonage, S., "Resistance to slimming: Adaptation or illusion", *Lancet,* 1975: 1: 733.

-Mindell, E., *Creating Your Personal Vitamin Plan*, Keats Publishing, New Canaan, CT, 1996, p. 52.

-Mindell, E., *What You Should Know About Herbs,* Keats Publishing, New Canaan, CT, 1996.

-Mokdad, A.H., Serdula, M.K., Dietz, W.H., et.al., "The spread of obesity epidemic in the United States, 1991-1998," Journal of American Medical Association, 1999, 282"(16): 1519-1522

-Morgan, B.L.G., Morgan R. *Hormones How They Affect Behavior, Metabolism, Growth, Development and Relationships,* The Body Press, Los Angeles CA, 1989.

-Mowrey, D.B., "Thermogenesis: The Whole Story," Let's Live Magazine, Los Angeles CA, Vol. 63, No. 11, 1995, p. 60-63.

-Mowrey, D., "Get Moving," The Energy Times, Long Beach, CA, 1:96:50-56.

-Muha. L., "Can You Escape Fat Fate?" Fitness Magazine, New York, NY: May 1997, p.121.

-Mulhsen. L., Rogers, J.Z., "Complementary and Alternative Modes of Therapy For the Treatment Of The Obese Patient," The Journal of The American Osteopathic Association, Vol. 99, No: , Part 2, October, 1999, p S8-S11.

-Natural Health Editors, *The 1996 Natural Health Handbook,* Natural Health Magazine, Brookline Village MA, 1996, p. 50.

-*Take the "2 Minute" Fiber Test,* Nature's Secret, Boulder, CO.

-*Naturopathic Hand Book of Herbal Formulas,* Herbal Research Publications, Ayer, MA, 1995, p. 12-13.

-"Negative Calorie Foods, Happy Healthy and Wealthy," Roy UT, (found on-line at www.happyheatlhyandwealthy.com/info/calorie.htm)

-Null, G., Null, S., *How To Get Rid of The Poisons In Your Body,* Prentice Hall Press, NY, 1977 p 168-169.

- "Obesity In America," Mayo Clinic Health Oasis, CNN.com, October 5, 2001

-Osman, J., *Thin From Within,* Hart Publishing Co., NY, 1976.

-Otto, J. H., *Modern Health,* Holt, Rinehart and Winston, NY, 1967.

-Parrado, P.A., Sad But True: The Late Century is a Culture of Obesity", Better Nutrition, Atlanta, GA., Feb., 1997, p.54-58.

-Passwater, R.A., "America's No. 1 Health Problem-Overweight but Undernourished: An Interview with Dr. Anthony Conte," Whole Foods Magazine, Plainfield, NJ, October 1996, p.48-57.

-Pasquaili, R., "Clinical Aspects of Ephendrine in The Treatment of Obesity," Journal of Obesity, 17.1 (1993): 565-568.

-Peeters, H. H., "Shortcut to Cutting Down Cholesterol," Medical Tribune, December, 22, 1974, p. 38E.

-Penn, F., "Cheat and Beat Your Metabolism" *Fitness Magazine,* New York, NY, May, 1997, p. 80-85.

-Pi-Sunyer, F.X., "The Fatting of America," Journal of The America Medical Association, (272), 7: 20:94.

-Pope, J., *The Last Five Pounds,* Simon And Schuster, NY, 1995.

-Ramazanov, Z., Suarez, M.M.B., *Effective Natural Stress and Weight Management Using Rhodiola Rosea and Rhododendrom Caucasicum*, ATN/Safe Goods Publishing, Sheffield, MA, 1999.

-Reed, B. P., *Nutrition: An Applied Science*, West Publishing, St. Paul, MN, 1980.

-Ritchason, J., *The Little Herb Encyclopedia*, Woodland Health Books, Pleasant Grove, UT, 1995.

-Rodgers, M., *Foods That Burn Fat* (Excerpts From his Book found on-line at www.livesmarter.com/burn-fat.html)

-Rogers, S., "How the Sick Get Sicker Quicker Without Nutritional Supplements," Let's Live 62, No. 1 (Jan, 1994): 44-47.

-Rosenbaum, M. E., "Chromium Polynicotinate: A Real Mouthful," Whole Foods, February 1990.

-Rudolph, M., "Solving The Supplement Puzzle," The Energy Times, Long Beach, CA, 1996, p. 29-35.

-Sahelian, R., *Melatonin Nature's Sleeping Pill*, Behappier Press, Marina Del Ray, CA, 1995.

-Saito, M., "Effect of soy peptides on energy metabolism in obese animals," Nutrition Science, 1991, (12): 91.

-Sandler, D., "How Do You Measure Up?" Oxygen Magzine, Hollywood, FL, Jan./Feb, 1990, p. 40.

-Santillo, H., *Food Enzymes, The Missing Link To Radiant Health*, Hohm Press, Prescott, AZ, 1987.

-Schulz, H. "Effects of Hypericum Extract On Sleep - EEG In Older Volunteers." The Journal of Geriatry, Psychiatry and Neurology, Oct. 1994, 7:S39-43.

-Sears, B., *Enter The Zone*, Harper and Collins, NY, 1995.

-Seaton, T.B., Welle, S.L., Warenko, M.K. Campbell, R.G., "Thermic Effect of Medium and Long Chain Triglycerides in Man," The American Journal of Clinical Nutrition, (44) 1986; 630-634.

-Shealy, N., *DHEA The Youth and Health Hormone*, Keats Publishing, New Canaan, CT, 1996, p. 44.

-Silverstone, T., et.al., "The Clinical Pharmacology of Appetite Supress ant Drugs," Internal Journal Obesity, 8.1 (1984): 23-33.

-Sonnenbichler, J., et al., "Influence of Silybin On The Synthesis of Macromolecules In Liver Cells" Proceedings of the International Bioflavonoid Symposiums, Munich, FGR: 1981, p. 477.

-Sparkman, D.R., "DHEA, The Magic Bullet For Targeting Fat Reduction," Muscular Development Magazine, Hollywood FL, Oct. 1996, p. 32-37.

-Stanko, R. T., et al., "Inhibition Of Lipid Accumulation And Enhancement Of Energy Expenditure By The Addition Of Pyruvate And Dihydroxyacetone To A Rat Diet," Metabolism 35:182-186; 1986.

-Starr, C., Taggart, R., *Biology: The Unity and Diversity of Life*, Wadsworth Publishing, NY, 1987.

-Sullivan, A. C., Hamilton, J. G., Miller, O. N., Wheatley, V. R. "Inhibition of Lipogenesis In Rat Liver by (-)Hydroscycitrate," Arch. Biochem. Biophys. 150:183-190, 1972.

-Sullivan, A. C. and Triscari, J. "Metabolic Regulation as a Control for Lipid Disorders. I., Influence of (-) Hydroxycitrate on Experimentally Induced obesity in the Rodent," Am. J. Clin. Nutr. 30:767-776, 1977.

-Sunderland, G. T., et al., "A double blind, Randomized Placebo-Controlled Trail of Hexopal In Primary Raynaud's Disease," Clinical Rheumarol; 7 (1988): 46-49.

-"Theraputic Foods Nutrition Council, Health Line," New York Hospital-Cornell Medical Center To Establish National Garlic Center, Vol. 2, Issue 5, New York, NY, Nov/Dec., 1994.

-Tomita, T., Yuasa, C., Ishimura, R. N., Ichihara, A., "Long Term Maintenance of Functional Rat Hepatocytes in Primary Culture by Additions of Pyruvate and Various Hormones," Biochimica et Biophysica ACTA 1243.3 (1995): 329-335.

-Twigg, S., *Love Food ... Lose Weight,* Penguin Publishing, NY, 1997

-"The Ultimate Diet Secret Blue Green Immortality," Health Watchers System, Scottsdale, AZ, 1996.

-Urberg, M., et al, "Hypocholesterolemie Effects of Nicotinic Acid And Chromium Supplementation," Journal of Family Practice, 27 (6) 603-606, 1988.

-Vanderhoek, J., el al., "Inhibition Of Fatty Acid Lipoxygenases By Onion And Garlic Oils. Evidence For The Mechanism By Which These Oils Inhibit Platelet Aggregation," Biochemical Pharmacology, 1980, 29, 3:169-173.

-Van Gaal, et al., "Explortory Study of Coenzyme Q10 in Obesity," Folkers and Yamura, Vol 4, 1984, p. 369-373.

-Van Gaal, L.F., Snyders, D., DeLeuw, L.H. Bekaert, J.L., "Anthropometric and Calormetric Evidence For The Protein Sparing Effects of a New Protein Supplemented Low Caloric Preparation," American Journal of Clinical Nutrition, 1985; 41: 540-544.

-Vahouny, G., Kritchevsky, D., *"Dietary Fiber," Health and Disease,* Plenum Press, NY, 1982.

-Vickery, D.M., *Life Plan For Your Health,* Addison Wesley, Reading MA, 1978.

-Wade, C., *Helping Your Health with Enzymes,* Parker Publishing Co. West Nyack, NY, 1966.

-Walker, M., "High Fiber Foods: Solid Facts Behind The Hype," Whole Foods, Plainfield, NJ, 10:90: 33-38.

-Ward, J. A., Hetzel, H. R., *Biology, Today and Tomorrow,* 2nd Ed., St. West Publishing Co., Paul, MN, 1984.

-Warmbrand, M., *The Encyclopedia of Health and Nutrition,* Pyramid Books, NY, 1962.

-Webster, D., *Acidophilus and Colon Health,* Hygeia Publishing, Cardiff, CA, 1991.

-"Weight-loss Drugs: The Next Generation," USA Today, Tuesday, Oct 14, 1997.

-Weil A., *Health and Healing*Houghton-Mifflin Company, Boston MA, 1995.

- "The Secret of 851 Oral Liquid Soy," Wheat Grass Express, Gainesville, FL, 1996.

-Wilson, A. C., et al., "Lecithin In Hyperlipidemia" American Journal of Clinical Nutrition, 119:496-501,1989.

-Wood, H.C., *Overfed But Undernourished,* Exposition Press, Inc., NY, 1959.

-Wojcick, J., et.al., "Clinical Evaluation of Lecithin as a Lipid Lowering Agent," Phytotherapy Res. 9, 1995.

-Wurtman, J. J., *Managing Your Mind and Mood Thru Food,* Rawson Associates, NY, 1986.

Other Titles from Safe Goods Publishing

All-Natural High Performance Diet	$ 7.95US $11.95CA
The Sugar Addict's Diet	$12.95US $19.95CA
Nutritional Leverage for Great Golf	$ 9.95US $14.95CA
Feeling Younger with Homeopathic HGH	$ 7.95US $11.95CA
The Secrets of Staying Young	$ 9.95US $14.95CA
Lower Cholesterol without Drugs	$ 6.95US $10.95CA
Super Nutrition for Dogs n' Cats	$ 9.95US $14.95CA
Macrobiotics for Americans	$ 7.95 US $11.95 CA

For a complete listing of books visit our website
www.safegoodspub.com
or call for a free catalog (888) 628-8731

order line: (888) NATURE-1

NOTES: